TELEMENTAL HEALTH

Telemental Health

What Every Student Needs to Know

Rosanne Nunnery, PhD and
Lisa McKenna, PhD, Editors

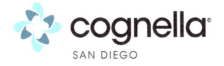

cognella®

SAN DIEGO

Bassim Hamadeh, CEO and Publisher
Amy Smith, Senior Project Editor
Abbey Hastings, Production Editor
Jess Estrella, Senior Graphic Designer
Kylie Bartolome, Licensing Coordinator
Ursina Kilburn, Interior Designer
Natalie Piccotti, Director of Marketing
Kassie Graves, Senior Vice President, Editorial
Jamie Giganti, Director of Academic Publishing

Cover image: Copyright © 2020 iStockphoto LP/Ivan Pantic.

Design images: Copyright © by UXWing.

Printed in the United States of America.

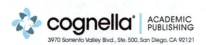

cognella® | ACADEMIC PUBLISHING

3970 Sorrento Valley Blvd., Ste. 500, San Diego, CA 92121

This book is dedicated to my husband, John Barrett, and children John, Alex, and Lillian. I love you. Thank you for encouraging me to take my creative ideas and be brave enough to contribute them to the world. Risks do have rewards.

—Rosanne

This book is dedicated to my sons, Austin, Ryan, and Brady, for making me strive to be better every day; to my soulmate, Kevin, for always being by my side; and to my parents and sister, Don, Betty, and Julie, for always believing in me. I love you all more than words can express!

—Lisa

Brief Contents

Detailed Contents

CHAPTER 3

Technical and Practical Considerations for Telemental Health   63

Nicole M. Arcuri Sanders

CHAPTER 4

Conducting Preliminary and Clinical Assessments in Telemental Health   81

Rosanne Nunnery and Ann Melvin

CHAPTER 5
Delivering Clinical Skills in a Telemental Health Setting   105

Lisa McKenna and Rosanne Nunnery

CHAPTER 6
Documentation and Billing in Telemental Health   133

Lisa Giovannelli

CHAPTER 7
Application of Telemental Health, Part 1: Young Children   155
Jen Green

CHAPTER 8
Application of Telemental Health, Part 2: Adolescents and Older Adults   173
Missy Fauser

CHAPTER 9

Application of Telemental Health, Part 3: Couples, Families, and Groups   193

Nicole M. Arcuri Sanders and Alisha Davis

CHAPTER 10

Application of Telemental Health, Part 4: Additional Areas of Specialization   215

Fredrick Dombrowski

CHAPTER 11

Counselor Self-Care in Telemental Health Practice 241

Kelly A. James

ACTIVE LEARNING

This book has interactive activities available to complement your reading.

Your instructor may have customized the selection of activities available for your unique course. Please check with your professor to verify whether your class will access this content through the Cognella Active Learning portal (http://active.cognella.com) or through your home learning management system.

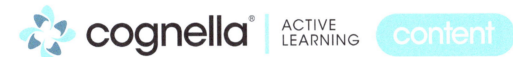 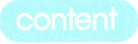

Preface

The motivation to write this book stems from our personal experiences as counselors and counselor educators, and our specific work serving clients in a telemental health setting. Over the last several years, there has been a growing trend for counselors to meet the needs of clients beyond the traditional face-to-face office setting by extending their reach remotely via video, phone, and/or chat sessions. With the global pandemic, state licensing boards expanded work with clients to telemental health so that clients could be served when stay-at-home orders were required. As counselor educators, we have seen the need for and benefits of distance services in the field of counseling for many years. We live in a world where individuals need flexibility and accessibility. Many universities and state licensure boards have implemented focused training and guidelines to help pre- and postgraduate counselors practice telemental health legally and ethically. As a result, our goal in writing this book is to help provide future counselors with varied tools to assist you with understanding what constitutes telemental health, skills necessary for this platform, assessment processes, laws and ethics, and application with varied populations. As you are the future of the helping profession, this book will help expand your knowledge so that you are better equipped to work with clients across different modalities.

Who This Book Is For

This book was written primarily for graduate-level students in counseling and related fields, although any helping professional new to providing telemental health services can certainly benefit. In our research on telemental health, we found that the available literature targeted licensed/credentialed practitioners. Our combined experience teaching graduate counseling students in online programs informed us that counselors in training would benefit greatly during their training from learning about telemental health. Preparing trainees to work in a tech-savvy culture where people are accustomed to engaging with others via computers and handheld devices will enhance their educational experience and marketability when applying for competitive fieldwork placements. This book is intended to be used as a supplemental book for graduate students in pre-practicum classes, interns in practicum, pre-licensed professionals, and professionals new to telemental health.

The information in this book is intended to be presented in a conversational and approachable manner. We hope you find the tone and delivery of the information engaging and supportive of your balance in adding an additional resource to your reading list. Each author was selected based on their specialization and professional experience. As you read, you will see some variation in terms across specializations (e.g., counselors versus therapists) and by different professionals (e.g., counselors in training versus students). Our professional identity is professional counseling, so this book aligns closely with the American Counseling Association's (ACA) ethical codes. We are confident that the material in this book is applicable to both professional counseling and related fields, and we encourage all readers to explore their specific ethical codes as they relate to the practice of telemental health.

Structure of the Book

This book offers 11 chapters that address varied aspects of telemental health work. The flow of the book begins by addressing historical aspects and then progresses to exploring ethical and legal considerations, technical and practical considerations, assessment, clinical skills, documentation and billing, work with specialized populations, and counselor self-care. Within many of the chapters you will find features such as case applications, personal reflection prompts and/or application activities, prompts to bookmark helpful websites, and excerpts from interviews with professional counselors in the field. Each author applies these varied activities in unique ways but seeks to help you apply the knowledge learned in the chapter to work with clients and your own self-reflection and growth, and to learn from others working in telemental health.

Contents of the Book

In Chapter 1, the history of telemental health is explored. We define common terms, abbreviations, and emoticons that are commonly used in telemental health practice. As the chapter unfolds, there is an articulation of the key benefits, potential challenges, and strategies to address the challenges within a telemental health practice. Finally, we provide information regarding additional training resources for counselors that would like to earn specific credentials in telemental health.

In Chapter 2, the authors identify relevant codes of ethics by examining, primarily, ACA's code and providing additional codes and resources relevant to telemental health across related professions. There is focus on federal and state laws that regulate telemental health counseling and supervision. When considering ethics, it is critical to consider an ethical decision-making process to navigate choices when ethical dilemmas emerge.

Chapter 3 focuses on technical and practical considerations for telemental health. Guidance is offered regarding consideration and application of ways to create a telemental health space that is professional and confidential.

Chapter 4 emphasizes the importance of integrating assessments in a telemental health setting. There is a description of the role of assessment in general, and then specifically on preliminary screening assessments and clinical assessments that are commonly used in telemental health. Initial screenings for appropriate fit for telemental health, biopsychosocial assessments, and crisis and suicide assessments are discussed, with a focus on how to navigate these digitally. Specific examples of assessments and how these can be adapted to the needs of your own work with clients are provided.

Chapter 5 delves into how clinical skills can be delivered effectively in a telemental health setting. It is imperative that foundational skills and relationship-building strategies translate into a telemental health environment. Ways to effectively identify problems and setting goals are discussed. A case example is provided and referenced throughout the chapter that offers visibility into how a counselor builds a relationship upon initial contact via a chat and continues to develop the relationship as counseling interventions and techniques unfold. Just as the beginning of the relationship is critical, so too is the understanding of how to effectively make referrals and progress to appropriate termination.

Chapter 6 extends the importance of work with clients to understanding the importance of documentation and billing in telemental health. Although trainees cannot bill prior to being licensed, having the knowledge of documentation needs specific to telemental health will prepare you for future documentation and what is needed for appropriate billing and reimbursement. Recording keeping and record maintenance, as well as examples of ways to appropriately do this, plus a case scenario, are covered to help increase competence with the process.

Chapter 7 begins part one of focusing on a specialized population, young children. This author addresses the importance of understanding the developmental aspects of young children. There are specific models and reflective activities that can be applied with young children in a telemental health setting. Pros and cons of working in telemental health are addressed along with ways to increase skills in this area to effectively apply interventions with young children.

Chapter 8 continues to focus on application and looks at telemental health practice with adolescent and older adult populations. Drawing on the author's extensive experience working with these populations, specific considerations that can support counselors in developing and maintaining rapport in a distance setting are addressed. This chapter provides creative techniques and examples that can be effectively applied in a telemental health platform.

Chapter 9 focuses on part 3 of the application to specialized populations, couples, families, and groups. These authors provide an overview of unique attributes of telemental health services. There is information regarding ethical implications, and case applications are provided to effectively apply specific skills and strategies when working with a couple, family, or group.

Chapter 10 focuses on part 4 of the application to specialized populations. This is not an exhaustive analysis but does explore individuals with intellectual disabilities, chronic pain, individuals in recovery, and LGBTQ+ populations. The author explores the benefits and limitations in using telemental health and unique needs for the populations identified. There is a focus on how to mitigate challenges and address them effectively by integrating resources to support effective telemental health implementation.

Chapter 11 is the final chapter that closes out the book with a discussion of the importance of self-care practices for telemental health practitioners. The author explores why self-care is important, addresses strategies for self-care specific to telemental health counselors, and then walks the reader through an example self-care plan.

Acknowledgments

Completing such a large project is a rewarding and sacrificial process. We (Rosanne and Lisa) would like to extend our appreciation to everyone reading this book. We prepared it for you and are grateful that there was an interest in and need for expanding your knowledge in telemental health. We would like to thank the publisher for reading our proposal and vision for creating a telemental health book for trainees that could be used as a supplement to guide their practice in an ever-growing technological world. To our stellar colleagues, thank you for contributing your time, energy, and creative skills to the completion of your chapters. It is such a privilege and an honor to have partnered with you on this project! We are also so grateful for the many brilliant and amazing colleagues who shared their perspectives and experiences providing telemental health services, and whose excerpts from interviews you will find throughout the book. To our families, we thank you for your love and support, especially since there were many long hours spent writing and editing. Without your continual encouragement from start to completion we would not have had the ability to complete this project.

CHAPTER 1

The Evolution of Telemental Health

Rosanne Nunnery and Lisa McKenna

Technology is best when it brings people together.

–Matt Mullenweg, Social Media Entrepreneur, Co-Founder of WordPress

Learning Objectives

After reading this chapter, you should be able to do the following:

1. Describe telemental health, including the history
2. Define common terms, abbreviations, and emoticons relevant to telemental health practice
3. Articulate key benefits, potential challenges, and success strategies associated with telemental health practice
4. Identify training resources for telemental health

Introduction

Telemental health practice has been gaining a lot of attention over the years, especially since the start of the global pandemic. Counselors have been advocating to policymakers for their services to be more accessible to clients, and telemental health is one advancement that can make this possible. As a graduate student, you may be curious how telemental health will impact your current training and future practice as a counselor. You may be asking, *How can my training translate in a telemental health setting? Will I be competent to work with clients on a digital platform? Is there anything I can do now, regardless of where I am in my training, to become better prepared?* In this book, our goal is to address these questions and more! First, let's take a closer look at how technology has already greatly influenced how we function in our daily lives.

In our digital and technologically advanced society, chances are that as a graduate student you have at least one electronic device that guides your daily activities. These devices are part of entertainment, socializing, shopping, working, dating, and studying. Take a moment and think about all the technology devices that you and/or people close to you use every day. In this list, you probably have included handheld devices such as cell phones and tablets, and computers of all shapes and sizes. These devices make technology accessible whether you are at home, in school, in your local community, or wherever you may travel. The following finding will likely not come as a surprise, but over a decade ago Lin (2010) identified cell phone use as the most widely used electronic device in the world, especially in Western society. More recently, the Pew Research Center (who tracks cell phone usage by age) indicated that over 90% of adults own a cell phone, with over 80% owning a smartphone (2021). That is a lot of lives impacted by instant access to information and available connections with others at their fingertips!

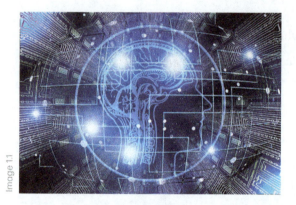

Image 1.1

As individuals, we use social media in part to communicate and engage with others and as a means of sharing information at a very rapid rate. This includes the use of social networking, blogging, micro blogging, wikis, social news, media sharing, opinions, reviews, ratings, and exploring topics (Duggan et al., 2015; Koukaras et al., 2020). Social networking platforms, such as Facebook, Instagram, Snapchat, and Twitter (among a few!), are one example of how technology has become a natural part of our daily experience (Duggan et al., 2015; Yu et al., 2018). Thinking beyond social connections, consider the ease of accessibility to almost any product, tutorial, or service. Can you imagine life without websites such as Amazon? eBay? Etsy? Any other companies that support your every product wish with a click?

BUILDING A VIRTUAL TELEMENTAL HEALTH TOOLBOX

We recommend that you take a moment now to create a **virtual telemental health toolbox** on your favorite web browser. After creating and naming your folder, explore the websites suggested for review throughout the chapter and decide which ones you'd like add to your toolbox. We'll flag the resources for you; stay on the lookout for the reminder "**Time to Bookmark!**"

Technology has also supported individuals with their personal and professional learning goals. Sometimes referred to as YouTube University, any tutorial on any subject is available 24/7. Formal educational institutions have also sought ways to expand their reach in order to keep up with the era of technology. For example, universities have used technology to support goals of increased enrollment and improve quality of instruction, teaching, and learning, and evaluation of data (Orr et al., 2018). Universities have been required to rethink their approach to instruction and learning from primarily synchronous face-to-face (Ft) to asynchronous (non-FtF) learning, or a combination of both methods, with an emphasis on the use of video platforms to connect students and faculty (Gloria & Uttal, 2020; Sommers-Flanagan, J. & Sommers-Flanagan, 2017). Prior to the COVID-19 pandemic, distance education had already begun to open opportunities for both traditional and nontraditional students. Since the pandemic, many traditional brick-and-mortar universities across the world were suddenly faced with the need to shift to online (Harrison, 2021; Moorhouse, 2020).

In the field of counselor education, universities have been expanding their offerings to fully online or hybrid platforms for their counseling programs over many years (ACES Technology Interest Network, 2017; Snow & Coker, 2020). This has created an opportunity for students to learn the necessary communication and counseling delivery skills needed within a digital context. Even if you are a student in a traditional higher education institution, technology skills are still important, and you likely are already integrating some technology in your training. Have you ever utilized an online discussion board? Online social networking group? These are advantageous to consider implementing either on your own with your peers, or through the assistance of your faculty. Whether at the beginning of your program of study, in a skills class, or toward the end of your program in your fieldwork experience (practicum and internship); you will likely be exposed to the concept of distance counseling or telemental health as the advancements in technology continue to grow.

VOICES FROM THE FIELD

What advice do you have for counseling students learning telemental health?

"My advice is to not fear it and not see it as something less than. On some level, I think it takes even more effort than an office setting. We are really face to face—microexpressions can be seen more clearly and clients tend to be more forthcoming as their own comfort level with technology makes it a more accessible platform. You get to see your clients in a way we never have before and I think there is great benefit in that."

–Melissa Lee-Tammeus, PhD, LMHC, Jacksonville, FL

"I tell students to be in a room that resembles a therapy office (not a bedroom), dress professionally, and remove any distractions. Video sessions might be a different platform, but the expectations are the same."

–Erin Pannell, PhD, LPC-S, RPT-S, Austin, Texas

"Continue the focus on building rapport first and foremost. Nothing works without the connection! This is the same with technology and in person. It does not matter which form the communication occurs in, if you cannot connect, nothing will work."

–Robin Switzer, PhD, LPC, St Louis, MO

A Look at the History of Telemental Health

The history of telehealth for professionals is not new. In fact, distant practice began with telemedicine. The prefix "tele" means distant, at a distance, or over a distance. This practice started in the medical field since patients were unable to meet in an office face-to-face due to factors such as distance to office, cost, and transportation challenges. Physicians were historically first to utilize telephones as a method to complete their work and to maintain patient contact and a continuum of care (Baumann & Scales, 2016; Nesbit, 2012). In the early 1920s Haukeland Hospital in Norway utilized radio links to diagnose and treat individuals (Nesbit, 2012). The first mention of any form of telemedicine in the literature specific to medical care came around 1950, with radiologists using video communication at the University of Nebraska (Field, 1996; Nesbit, 2012). Telepsychiatry use was also used in the state of Nebraska at a psychiatric institute where videoconferencing served as a tool for psychiatrists' medical training and to conduct group and other long-term therapies, including medication maintenance. Typically, these methods were utilized for those who lived in doctor-deficient locations. The American Psychiatric Association (APA) reports that in the late 1960s Massachusetts General Hospital engaged in telepsychiatry in a clinic at Logan airport, and this practice continued and became more common through the 70s and 80s (Von Hafften, n.d.). Telephone crisis counseling was started in London in the early 50s, with expansion into the United States in the 70s due to ease of access for those who had immediate need for intervention (Hornblow, 1986). This set the pace for common practice use in health care by connecting with individuals via the telephone and then eventually video conferencing, and many agencies developed practice guidelines (Von Hafften, n.d.). As technology has continued to advance, these guidelines (which will be discussed in more depth in a later chapter) have expanded. Telepsychiatry can provide a natural transition into mental health practice, as clients can be served via telemental health in the professional counseling field and related helping professions.

From the 1990s to today, telemental health has evolved to become common practice. This has been possible via the use of advances in technology, including advanced audio and video software, chat availability, emails, online therapy systems, virtual reality, and encryption capabilities to secure privacy for clients (Barnett & Scheetz, 2003; Rispoli & Machalicek, 2020). Originally many counselors utilized emerging platforms such as Skype to conduct distant sessions (Gilbertson, 2020). However, initially the reliability of these platforms was in question. Over time, improvements with technology and advancements in video conferencing and internet capabilities resulted in these platforms becoming more reliable and dependable. As the capabilities emerged, mental health professionals and those who were served began to consider the feasibility and likelihood of providing or receiving services in these varied contexts.

With the COVID-19 pandemic, the emergence of platforms that hire licensed professionals to service clients who want to receive mental health services has expanded. These platforms are companies that are owned by a third party and contract with counselors (with most receiving an hourly rate). These platforms can be accessed via online browsers and smartphone apps that are easily accessible, which both meets and increases the large demand for telemental health services around the world.

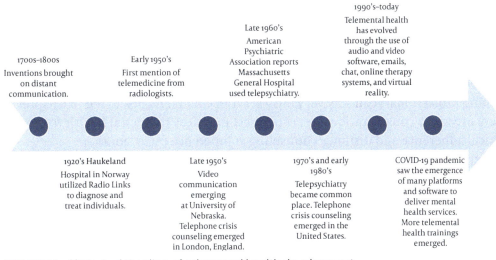

FIGURE 1.1   Historical timeline of telemental health development.

Working With Telemental Health Platforms

Once you are independently licensed, you can consider offering your services through one of these platforms. At that time, you will want to have a good idea of what the process looks like and what each platform offers, so do your homework before applying!

At the time of this writing, typically counselors apply to the companies by indicating their interest on their website or app. Oftentimes, a resume or curriculum vitae is requested. If selected for an interview, a representative from that company will conduct an interview and outline the expectations of working with the platform, including maintenance of licensure and abiding by the laws of your specific state. If hired, there is an expectation to retain licensure. Due to lack of reciprocity with licensure, it is imperative that the licensed professional only serve clients within their licensure parameters. Prior to beginning work for the company, specific documents can be uploaded for client review before they agree to work with you and you accept them as a client. These documents might include an informed consent, assessment questions, and your welcome message. Some of the platforms are subscription (often monthly) based for unlimited video, talk, or chat, while others have an insurance billing option and sessions might be 30 or 50 minutes. Potential clients complete a questionnaire to assist the company team with matching the client to the professional, and then the professional reviews the information and can accept or decline the client but must provide rationale (e.g., referral to another source based on areas of expertise). Although there are steps to get started and expectations for each company, the professional can make their own schedule and hours as well choose to be open to new clients. This is beneficial, especially for professionals balancing multiple responsibilities, other employment, or who have a full caseload. After services are rendered, contractors will receive a weekly or a monthly check from the clocked hours completed. As an independent contractor, there is flexibility in working a few hours a week or up to a full-time case load. Due to the broad range of clients that can be served, multiple matchings can happen every day. With all the available options, helping professionals can stay very busy serving clients! As discussed in Chapter 2, there are many considerations to ensure best practices in mental health to ensure ethical adherence and distance counseling competence (ACA, 2014).

There are many options today, with more continuing to emerge, for companies that hire counselors to provide telemental health practice via their platform. Examples of companies in the market today include Better Help, Talk Space, Calmerry, NOcd, Online-therapy.com, Pride Counseling, and AbleTo. When you are exploring possible platforms, it is important to understand what benefits are available to both the counselor and the client and the expected experience for both (e.g., understanding the fee structure). Following are some questions you may want to consider while you are researching options. Feel free to copy/print this form and fill it in for each company you research. Confirming the date you reviewed the company is helpful, as companies often change and you want current information before making any career/referral decisions.

TABLE 1.1 **Research for Telemental Health Platforms**

Company Platform: _____

Date: _____

Questions to Consider	Answer
MONETARY	
What is the compensation rate for professional counselors?	
Are benefits a possibility?	
Does the platform provide compensation for no-show clients?	
What is the fee structure for clients?	
TECHNICAL	
Is the platform HIPPAA compliant?	
Does the platform have end-to-end encryption?	
Is a business associate's agreement completed on behalf of the professional?	
Is a website made available to the counselor that can be personalized?	
EXPERIENTIAL	
Are client/counselors matched based on expertise/preferences?	
What services are available to clients through the platform (e.g., video, chat, email, phone, mobile app capabilities, scheduling supports such as reminders and access to make/change appointments, etc.)?	
Does the platform offer the counselor forms/documents/screening instruments to use and/or personalize?	
Can the counselor upload their own documents?	
What flexibility is offered the counselor in accepting/adding clients?	

(Continued)

Questions to Consider	Answer
What flexibility is offered the client in changing counselors?	
Can the client use health insurance directly with this platform?	
How does the platform support the emergency/crisis management process?	
OTHER (Add additional questions and/or notes)	

Just as there are platforms designed to hire professionals to work as independent contractors, there are many companies that offer telemental health software platforms to support independent practitioners for use in their own clinical practice. Current examples of these companies include Therapy Notes, Simply Practice, and EHR. This type of service is ideal for creating an online presence where potential clients can locate licensed professionals along with assist with maintaining records, billing capabilities, and encrypted software for confidential telemental health practice. These types of programs can be cloud based or an installed software program. It can be quite confusing to know the difference between the two:

> *Cloud-based programs*: "Cloud computing is the delivery of computing services— including servers, storage, databases, networking, software, analytics, and intelligence over the Internet ("the cloud") to offer faster innovation, flexible resources, and economies of scale" (Ranger, 2022, para. 1).
>
> *Installed software programs*: A program that is downloaded to a computer. This requires the purchase of the software, the initial cost to install on one or multiple computers, and ongoing maintenance as new versions emerge. They do not require the internet to access.

Typically, cloud-based programs are easier and more cost effective, while installed programs have a higher upfront and maintenance cost. The choice of which type of program is dependent on the type of practice, whether solo practice, group practice, or a large agency. Having a software program is typically beneficial for larger practices, whereas cloud-based programs are ideal for independent practice. Most of the platforms are moving toward being cloud based, although installed programs offer resources as well.

When comparing services offered, there is variation between what is offered to the practitioner and the client. Platforms offer practitioners the capability for a small practice in an outpatient or inpatient/residential arena with the capability of a small or larger scale of practitioners. Most of the providers offer electronic records and billing services, scheduling accessibility, the processing of credit cards, secure record storage, and either a single or multiple provider program. Depending on the services utilized, there is access to assessments, treatment planning, progress notes, visits/communication tracking, and mobile app availability. Additionally, practitioners can often create their own documents to be uploaded on the platform. These same platforms provide clients access to a client portal, where they can schedule/cancel appointments (and receive reminder notices), access forms and resources, use a mobile app to contact a practitioner, and use electronic billing.

TIME TO BOOKMARK!

For more information on comparing software platforms for telemental health, see https://telementalhealthcomparisons.com/

The Language of Technology

With the growth of telemental health, it has become imperative to consider how it is defined. At a broad level, telemental health can be defined as providing mental health services while a client and the practitioner are located in two different physical locations and communicate via the use of electronic means. The Health Resources and Services Administration (HRSA, n.d.) of the U.S. Department of Health and Human Services (HHS) defines telehealth as "the use of electronic information and telecommunications technologies to support and promote long-distance clinical health care, patient and professional health related education, and public health and health information" (para. 1).

A similar and expanded definition of telehealth is provided by the World Health Organization (WHO, 2010):

> The delivery of health care services, where distance is a critical factor, by all health care professionals using information and communication technologies, for the exchange of valid information for diagnosis, treatment, and prevention of disease and injuries, research and evaluation, and for the continuing education of health care providers, in all the interests of advancing the health of individuals and their communities. (p. 3)

Along with merely understanding how telemental health is defined, it is important to understand the language associated with delivery of telemental health services. Also, as a telemental health provider you will likely see and use common acronyms and emoticons to help personalize and humanize chat/text messaging. Table 1.2 reviews some common terms, Table 1.3 acronyms, and Table 1.4 emoticons.

TABLE 1.2 Common Terminology of Telemental Health Practice

Term	Definition
Synchronous	Working together at the same time; real-time communication that is heard at the time it is spoken; comments between communicators is relayed immediately. *Examples: Video session or phone session*
Asynchronous	Communication is when information is processed with a time lag; comments between communicators are delayed and dependent on when the parties are in the online format and see the written or audio correspondence. *Examples: Emails, online messaging*
Originating site	The location of the client when telemental health services are used. This can be at a home on a computer or other smart device or in the office of a telemental health remote clinic.
Distant site	The location the counselor is offering the mental health counseling services by remote means to the originating site of the client.
Client portal	A secure internet sign-on that allows clients to contact, via message or email, their provider with a time lag. Clients can complete homework, review documentation and records, and set up appointments.
Store and forward	The process of collecting information from a client and uploading or sending the information electronically for the distant provider to review at another time. This might include demographic data, medical records, homework assignments, images, and labs/other reports.
Business associate agreement	A written document that outlines the specific arrangement and responsibilities between two parties to maintain protected health information.

TABLE 1.3   **Common Acronyms**

AFK	Away from keyboard
BBFN	Bye bye for now
BFN	Bye for now
BRB	Be right back
BTT	Back to topic
BTW	By the way
C&P	Copy and paste
CTN	Can't talk now
CU	See you
HTH	Hope this helps
IDK	I don't know
IIRC	If I recall/remember correctly
IMO	In my opinion
IOW	In other words
LMK	Let me know
LOL	Laughing out loud
NP	No problem
NRP	No reply necessary
OMW	On my way
OT	Off topic
SFLR	Sorry for late reply
TTYL	Talk to you later
TIA	Thanks in advance
TQ	Thank you
TYT	Take your time

(Continued)

TYVM	Thank you very much
WFM	Works for me
YMMD	You made my day

Note: Adapted from https://www.smart-words.org/abbreviations/internet-acronyms.png.

TABLE 1.4   **Sample Common Emoticons**

Emotion/Behavior	Manual Entry	Image (may vary by device)
Smile	:-)	😊
Sad	:-(	😞
Wink	;-)	😉
Cool	B-)	😎
Worried	:-s	😖
Surprise	:-O	😵
Laughing	:-))	😂
Big grin	:-D	😄

As more counselors and clients engage in the practice of telemental health service delivery, we become more aware of needs, benefits, potential challenges, and solutions to promote best practice.

VOICES FROM THE FIELD

What is the future of telemental health practice?

"I believe telemental health is here to stay and is a great way to reach vulnerable populations. We found in our area this service reached many more in rural settings that would not typically make a trip in town for counseling."

-Jeff McCarthy, PhD, LCPC, NCC, Ellsworth, ME

"Telemental health will become a consistent delivery system for mental health counseling. I think counseling needs to advocate for more infrastructure for WIFI access and connectivity. This is especially needed in rural areas."

-Cheryl Welch, PhD, LPC, RN, Florence, WI

"Telemental health is the silver lining on the dark cloud of Covid-19. It has made counseling more accessible to clients. It has made counseling also more accessible to counselors. And, it has made more job opportunities available to counselors!"

-Jennifer Meador, MS, LPC, ADC, NCC, CCTP, BC-TMH, Demopolis, Alabama

The Need for Telemental Health Practice

There is a high demand for mental health care and not enough service providers to meet this demand (Kaiser Family Foundation, 2018). The words of supply and demand often conjure up the idea of economics class or mathematics. Although some helping professionals enjoy mathematics and statistics along with watching the stock market as investments go up and down, the idea of supply and demand as a counselor may seem quite foreign. However, as future counseling professionals, supply and demand will be the driving force for employment, and while it may be uncomfortable for some who enter helping professions to focus on finances, you do want to have a thriving practice! Not only is there a great need to focus on your own personal and professional needs, but our world also needs professionals to service them due to the high rate of mental health needs. The WHO emphasizes that mental health care must be a top priority and should be included in any goal planning, with significant investment in prevention and intervention with mental health diagnoses. The WHO (n.d.) recognizes that since 2017 there has been a 13% increase in mental health and substance use disorders, and in their 2019 initiative they focused on plans to increase affordability, quality, and accessible coverage for mental health needs around the world. With an increase in mental health care accessibility, there will be a larger supply and demand for mental health services and an almost unlimited supply of folks needing services.

When looking at the economic definition of the word *demand* there is a clear distinction that it is a desire and a want by purchasers, consumers, or others for a particular commodity with authority (Merriam-Webster, n.d.). As noted earlier, the WHO desires to expand access to mental health around the world. This means that the possibility of telemental health is far reaching to many different populations. This includes those with limited mobility or potentially those who are homebound, especially due to illness or required quarantine. Individuals with medical conditions, acute or chronic diagnoses, or those who are caretakers, need a venue to access mental health treatment. Other barriers to treatment that telemental health can help to bridge include lack of reliable transportation and lower financial resources that may hinder individuals' ability to receive services. Many community mental health agencies sought to reduce this gap by doing home-based therapy, but with advancements with technology, these visits can be successfully done in their own home while the helping professional is at another location. With the cost of living on the rise, there is a need for both people in two-partner homes to work (Statista, 2022), and there is an increasing strain on single parents, the elderly, and shift workers, resulting in scheduling conflicts. Telemental health provides access to different dates, times, and hours so that a broader range of clients can be served. With consideration of the urban versus rural environments, where helping professionals are limited and may actually be related or personally know the helping professionals, telemental health offers confidentiality of services. As noted in the history of telemental health, many folks of all ages prefer technological mediums due to the ease of sending/receiving messages, whether in real time or asynchronously. There is an almost unlimited supply of clients seeking telehealth services if practitioners are trained effectively (Usher-Pines et al., 2020).

Benefits of Telemental Health

When reviewing the literature on the benefits of telemental health, common areas emerge as benefits: accessibility, reduction of stigma, convenience, and cost effectiveness (Arafat et al., 2021; Howard et al., 2018; Usher-Pines et al., 2020). Other benefits of telemental health include the following:

Benefits to Client

- ☑ Accessibility of services and often more counselors from which clients may choose
- ☑ Often more affordable
- ☑ Various mediums of use for clients (video, audio, chat, email)
- ☑ Clients often feel less inhibition and more comfort being in their own space
- ☑ Clients may be more willing to reveal traumatic events via telemental health
- ☑ Clients have a greater sense of control

Benefits to Counselor

- ✅ Counselors can observe client in their natural environment
- ✅ Rapport building is easier for some when in their own environment
- ✅ Cost of overhead for counselors is lower
- ✅ Increased ability to offer services when offices may not be open

VOICES FROM THE FIELD

What are some benefits you have experienced with telemental health practice?

"Personal benefits are the freedom that telehealth provides by being home, being able to go outside in between sessions, and if I have a break, I can take care of things at my home. For clients, they have commented on the benefit of not having to drive to my office, wait in the lobby, and then have to drive back. They like not having to take two hours off during the day. Since I mainly do EMDR therapy, clients have indicated that they could not tell the difference of using the electronic tappers or doing manual tapping at home. The EMDR therapy was still as effective, which is a huge benefit. Another benefit is that I am licensed in Oklahoma and Texas, so I have a larger client base being licensed in multiple states. I have many clients who seek my services specifically because I specialize in EMDR therapy and trauma, and with telehealth they are able to use my services even living in a different state."

–Kelly James, PhD, LPC, NCC, Tulsa, Oklahoma

"It is remarkable, but I find the clients are so much more open to sharing some of the most intimate details without the fear of being judged. The conversations I have with clients are so much more enlightening and profound because they are in their own environment and feel safe to share their thoughts. As I think about it, I can see how it is very intimidating for a client to sit in a counselor's office. The counselor's office sometimes lends itself to an unintentional power differential because it is the counselor's space and not the client's space. Telemental health balances that perceived power differential and makes the experience for the client much more collaborative."

–Alice Crawford, PhD, LCPC, Carpentersville, IL

"A major benefit is safely conducting meaningful sessions. Given quarantine restrictions and other concerns, telemental health became the only practical solution. So, it provided much-needed services to those in need without skipping a beat. Other practical benefits came about through saving time, being convenient, et cetera. For example, by saving time in transporting to and from the clinic, more time could be spent developing counselors, gathering more resources for clients, and most everything else."

– Matt Glowiak, PhD, LCPC, CAADC, NCC, Bolingbrook, IL

Additional Benefits to Both Client and Counselor

- ☑ More options regarding availability for sessions
- ☑ Online exchanges can be saved and reviewed by the client and counselor

What are the potential challenges of telemental health? It is natural to have some apprehension about what is involved and how the process would work from both the counselor and client's perspective. Potential challenges include the fear of the public not being receptive, communication barriers, lack of training and technical knowledge, less efficiency, administrative strongholds such as laws and insurance, and the maintenance and distribution of confidential information (Arafat et al., 2021; Caver et al., 2019; Hjelm, 2005; Usher-Pines, et al., 2020). Table 1.5 provides a summary of potential challenges and strategies for effectively serving clients via telemental health. (Many of these potential challenges will be discussed in more detail in later chapters.)

TABLE 1.5 **Potential Challenges of Telemental Health and Helpful Solutions**

Potential Challenges	Helpful Strategies
Difficulty with risk assessment and intervening during a crisis.	Before starting with a client, counselors should complete a screening tool and develop a safety plan with the client.
Protecting health information and confidentiality may be more of a challenge.	This challenge can be averted by utilizing a program or company where all communication and documents are secured and compliant with the Health Insurance Portability and Accountability Act (HIPAA) and the Health Information Technology for Economic and Clinical Health Act (HITECH). Ask any company utilized for a business associate's agreement between the counselor and the company or platform.
Counselor/client could become too relaxed or client might present differently online.	It is important to lay out the expectations of the type of session, the setting of the session, and the professionalism expected from you and the client. This should be in the informed consent document.
Consideration of less therapeutic impact when compared to same location practice.	Multiple researchers comparing telemental health and traditional practice indicated that there is at least an equal and sometimes greater impact via telemental health.
Technical problems or poor knowledge and skill can interfere with sessions and counselor–client relationships.	Prior to working with a client, use a screening tool that assesses fit for online counseling along with technology knowledge. This includes exploring ways to mitigate when there is a power outage or breakdown in communication.

May miss cultural diversity needs of a client.	Cultural diversity should be addressed in the biopsychosocial assessment. It is recommended that an additional cultural assessment is completed so that cultural factors can be part of the treatment process from intake to termination of treatment.
Some clients struggle with rapport building in a distant setting.	Rapport building is difficult no matter the setting. The counselor must utilize the basic foundational skills to establish and maintain rapport.
Written language could be misinterpreted by a client.	Misinterpretation can happen via the written word or verbally. That makes it critical to answer the ongoing question "Am I interpreting or understanding this correctly?"
Potential for quickly stopping counseling without notice or seeing multiple counselors.	The informed consent should outline the policy of having one counselor at a time and encouraging progress with termination. However, just as in a traditional setting, clients have the right to leave treatment at any time and to change counselors.
Technology may lead to the client feeling less in control.	People are very accustomed to technology, and if seeking help via telemental health they are likely to not have a sense of being out of control but rather more in control.
Recording keeping and billing uncertainty by clients and counselors.	Whether the counselor is a contractor or works as an independent practitioner, billing and payment issues are addressed upfront before sessions begin.

As you progress in your training and become more experienced, you may come across additional challenge points. When this happens, your clinical supervisor will be a tremendous resource for you.

Telemental Health Training Emergence

As previously discussed, the historical emergence of telemedicine, telepsychiatry, and now telemental health has a rich history starting in the 1950s. With the growth of this practice, there were many organizations, training programs, and governing agencies that either created protocols for training or had pop-up training opportunities both in person and online. One pioneer in telemental health training is the Veterans Affairs (VA) health care system, where there is research dating back to 2002 regarding veterans involved in telemental health counseling (U.S. Department of Veterans Affairs, 2018). This resulted in the expansion of training for helping professionals to be well equipped to service the community. Caver et al. (2019) noted that between 2006 and 2015 there were over 12,000 VA mental health providers that have successfully completed their

TIME TO BOOKMARK!

While not an exhaustive list, the associations in Table 1.6 are some examples with helpful information that can be found online.

TABLE 1.6 **Helpful Associations/Agencies for Telemental Health Resources**

Association	For Further Information
American Telehealth Association	https://www.americantelemed.org/community/telemental-health/
The American Telemedicine Association, Telemental Health Special Interest Group Division	https://www.americantelemed.org/community/telemental-health/
The International Society for Telemedicine & eHealth	https://www.isfteh.org/
Health Resources and Services Administration: The Office for the Advancement of Telehealth (OAT)	https://www.hrsa.gov/rural-health/telehealth
Telehealth Resource Centers	https://telehealthresourcecenter.org/
American Counseling Association: Telebehavioral Health Information and Counselors in Health Care	https://www.counseling.org/knowledge-center/mental-health-resources/trauma-disaster/telehealth-information-and-counselors-in-health-care
American Mental Health Counselors Association: Telehealth Resources	https://www.amhca.org/publications/practiceguidelines/coronavirus/telehealth

web-based telemental health training at varied levels, depending on the specific helping professional. In 2010, the VA established the National TeleMental Health Center—a national effort to have a long reach to serve veterans with mental health needs (U.S. Department of Veterans Affairs, 2018).

When delving outside the VA system, there are many training opportunities for graduate students and future LPCs to gain more knowledge regarding telemental health. Having effective and available training can increase knowledge and close the barriers to individuals seeking services (Gonzalez et al., 2018).

When the COVID-19 pandemic engulfed the world, many countries required quarantine, which changed the landscape of trainees and the needs of both practitioners and those being served (Costa et al., 2021; Siedner et al., 2020). As a result, the opportunities to connect across online associations and training institutions have grown, including worldwide and local opportunities.

Why Should Graduate Counseling Students Train in Telemental Health Now?

Current resources tend to focus on supporting the credentialed, fully licensed practitioner to transition from traditional live counseling practice to include telemental health in their work. There has not been a lot of attention given to the students preparing to work with clients in fieldwork, perhaps in a telemental health setting or following graduation. As more clients (and students!) need to enhance remote abilities for services, it is of utmost importance that students are prepared to work with clients in both live and telemental health settings.

The need to prepare students to understand the impact of technology on the field of counseling has been in place for several years. The Council for Accreditation of Counseling and Related Education Programs (CACREP, 2016) has included specific standards that counseling programs must address in the curriculum. However, programs have the option of addressing these standards either from a knowledge standpoint (e.g., traditional academic assignments like a paper or a quiz) or as a skills activity (e.g., hands-on, applied activities that are assessed). While having the knowledge base of technology's influence on counseling practice is essential, students will be better positioned for fieldwork opportunities and postgraduate supervised clinical work, having had more direct training and experience in telemental health.

2016 CACREP STANDARDS RELEVANT TO TECHNOLOGY

Section 2.F.1.j: Technology's impact on the counseling profession

Section 2.F.5.d: Ethical and culturally relevant strategies for establishing and maintaining in-person and technology-assisted relationships

Section 2.F.5.e: The impact of technology on the counseling process

Section 6.B.2.g (Doctoral Standard): Modalities of clinical supervision and the use of technology

During the global pandemic starting in 2020, many students who were already engaged in supervised clinical practice found themselves quickly searching for available training opportunities so that they could competently continue service to clients and their academic progress. During this time, many companies that specialize in offering continuing education courses and training platforms made available telemental health training. As of the time of this writing, many schools and programs have partnered with established companies to offer training to their students and faculty. It is encouraged that you explore if a telemental health training option is available through your institution. If it is, great! Take it as soon as you are able so that you complete the training (ideally) in advance of securing a fieldwork placement (this will also make you more marketable to potential sites!). If it is not, we encourage you to seek out training on your own. You can also advocate for this need to your program's department faculty and leaders to support other students in need of telemental health training.

Veronica Avedician: Graduate Student, Capella University
Counseling Intern, Clearbrook
Arlington Heights, IL

Entering practicum and internship as a graduate student is stressful enough, let alone during a pandemic. Luckily, I had a great professor and mentor that helped offer some tips to guide me through the process. Ultimately though, it would still be left to me to find a site. My professor gave me one valuable piece of advice: to treat this situation the same as I would for a job, trying to set up an interview. I reached out to several counseling sites and was able to set up a Zoom interview with them. I believe it was the ability to see one another that helped me secure my internship.

When I met with my site supervisor, she advised me that most of the clients I would be meeting with would be through Zoom and depending on the State mitigations during the pandemic; there might be opportunities for face-to-face sessions. Still, I could not fathom the idea of not seeing a client face-to-face and still feeling like I was an effective counselor.

The populations I served and continue to serve at this site are individuals with intellectual and developmental disabilities (IDD). Since beginning my internship, about half of the clients I see are telemental health appointments using Zoom. The remaining portion of my clients I see in-person. There have been many benefits to using telemental health as far as convenience and ease of the technology. Access to telemental health has made counseling more readily available to our clients. However, the challenges that I have experienced have a lot to do with my ability as a counselor to ensure that I help establish a strong rapport with my clients using this technology. Ethical and legal considerations are important because when consulting with a client, we need to ensure that our clients have sessions with complete and total privacy for confidentiality. As a counseling student, it has been essential to ensure that my surroundings are secure and private during these sessions. I am also mindful that I do not cross any personal boundaries that might hinder our client/counselor relationship during the sessions.

What Is the Official BC-TMH Credential?

You may be seeing more signature lines from professional counselors, including the letters BC-TMH (board-certified telemental health provider). This credential is available to licensed practitioners through the Center for Credentialing and Education (CCE). According to the CCE Board Certified-Telemental Health Professional Credential Eligibility Policy (2021):

> The Center for Credentialing & Education (CCE) administers a rigorous, examination-based, professional credential program for telemental health specialization recognition—designated as the CCE Board Certified-Telemental Health (BC-TMH) Program. Those individuals who wish to be granted the BC-TMH credential must demonstrate that they have achieved state licensure or national certification as a counselor or other licensed, behavioral, or mental health professional. Additionally, qualified applicants must meet specific educational requirements related to a professional specialization in telemental health services, and successfully complete an examination to assess content knowledge to satisfy the requirements of this Program. (p. 1)

The CCE provides formal credentialing for distance work called the board certified-telemental health counselor credential (BC-TMH). To become credentialed, there are specific requirements and training programs recommended by their organization. They highlight and endorse two online programs as of 2021: Star Telehealth and Telehealth Certification Institute. The CCE requires the following nine core areas that are included in the approved training programs:

- Introduction to TeleMental Health
- Presentation Skills for TeleMental Health

TIME TO BOOKMARK!

For more information on this credential, please see the following websites:

CCE: https://www.cce-global.org/credentialing/bctmh

Star Telehealth: http://www.startelehealth.org/certificates-and-credentials

Telehealth Certification Institute: https://www.telementalhealthtraining.com/bc-tmh

- HIPAA Compliance for TeleMental Health
- Best Practices in Video TeleMental Health
- Crisis Planning & Protocols in Video TeleMental Health

- Choosing and Using Technology in TeleMental Health
- Orienting Clients/Patients to TeleMental Health
- Direct-to-Consumer TeleMental Health
- TeleMental Health Settings and Care Coordination

Chapter Summary

The history of telemental health reaches far back to the 1700s when inventors began discovering ways to expand communication. In the early and mid-20th century, medical doctors, seeking innovative ways to better serve their patients, found a need to reach beyond their current location using radio waves and video communication. As mental health needs were recognized within society and more psychiatric units emerged, telepsychiatry was sparked into the 1960s, and the trend in mental health needs from a medical, wellness, and evidence-based treatment perspective expanded as technology grew.

You learned about the increase in demand for telemental health services via a distance format and were provided examples of companies using telemental health and how those programs operate via cloud-based and installed software programs. There are varied ways to engage with clients in a distant format, which creates a challenge with understanding the language of technology, common terms used in the field, acronyms, and emoticons that all foster communication between counselor and client.

There are many benefits and some challenges that can be mitigated by a counselor-in-training's willingness to seek supervision, get applicable training, and maintain involvement in professional associations at the student level. Just as you are reading this book, more software is being developed and more training opportunities are emerging for supervisory and postgraduate telemental health work. At this point, you may be questioning your ability to not only learn new skills but deliver them in multiple settings. It is natural and expected to have these feelings; we assure you that you are not alone!

Working as a helping professional is an artful journey with beautiful strokes that slowly unfold to create a complete picture of a competent helping professional. This takes education, practice, openness to growth, and ongoing self-reflection and self-awareness. The choice of becoming a helping professional is drawn from many different influences in your life due to your experiences and personality characteristics. You have likely been encouraged to serve others due to your natural ability to be helpful to others within your family and community. Perhaps you have even taken an assessment that indicated a high likelihood a helping profession was in your wheelhouse and would be a natural transition to pursue as a career. Skillful behavior, regardless of the setting in which you practice, takes an investment of time with training, experience, and patience. There is no prescription for perfection but rather the need to be your authentic self and practice ethically and empathically with your clients. Part of gaining competence to practice is recognizing that the helping profession changes just as our society grows and changes. Not only do clientele's needs change, but the way in which services are delivered also changes. So, when choosing a helping professional in this digital age, it is important to not choose a career based on the method or format of delivering skills but to base it on the ability to gain competence to practice the skills no matter what setting or format. As society and technology continue to be more interdependent, the time is ripe to further your skill set and expand your reach to future clients!

PERSONAL REFLECTION ACTIVITY

Whether you are a new student, in the middle of your program, or already engaged in fieldwork, take this opportunity to consider some questions:

1. Right now, reflect on where you are in your training.

    a.   Why are you seeking training as a counselor/therapist?
    b.   What motivated you to start your program?
    c.   What personal strengths do you have to meet your goal?
    d.   Where are your continued areas for growth, and do you have a plan in place to support you?

2. Now consider practicing in a telemental health setting. How does this vision influence any of your previous responses?

    Journal your thoughts, and revisit to further reflect on your motivation and progress as you continue in your training.

References

ACES Technology Interest Network. (2017, May). *Guidelines for distance education.* https://www.nbcc.org/Assets/COVID/ACESGuidelinesforOnlineLearninginCounselorEducation.pdf

American Counseling Association. (2014). *Code of ethics.* Author.

Arafat, M., Zaman, S., & Hawlader, M. (2021). Telemedicine improves mental health in COVID-19 pandemic. *Journal of Global Health, 11*(03004), 1–4.

Barnett, J. E., & Scheetz, K. (2003). Technological advances and telehealth: Ethics, law, and the practice of psychotherapy. *Psychotherapy: Theory, Research, Practice, Training, 40*(1–2), 86–93. https://doi.org/10.1037/0033-3204.40.1–2.86

Baumann, P., & Scales. T. (2016). History of information communication technology and telehealth. *Academy of Business Research Journal, 3,* 48–52. https://go.openathens.net/

redirector/liberty.edu?url=https://www.proquest.com/scholarly-journals/history-information-communication-technology/docview/1863562170/se-2?accountid=12085

Caver, K. A., Shearer, E. M., Burks, D. J., Perry, K., Paul, N. F., McGinn, M. M., & Felker, B. L. (2020). Telemental health training in the Veterans Administration Puget Sound Health Care System. *Journal of Clinical Psychology, 76*(6), 1108–1124. https://doi.org/10.1002/jclp.22797

Center for Credentialing and Education. (2021, February 18). *Board Certified-Telemental Health Professional Credential Eligibility Policy* https://www.cce-global.org/Assets/BCTMH/bc-tmh_professional_credential_eligibility_policy.pdf

Costa, M., Reis, G., Pavlo, A., Bellamy, C., Ponte, K., & Davidson, L. (2021). Tele-mental health utilization among people with mental illness to access care during the COVID-19 pandemic. *Community Mental Health Journal, 57*(4), 720–726.

Council for Accreditation of Counseling and Related Educational Programs (CACREP) (2016). www.cacrep.org

Duggan, A. M., Ellison, N.B., Lampe, C., Lenhar, A., & Madden, M. (2015). *Social media update 2014.* Pew Research Center. https://media.myworshiptimes22.com/wp-content/uploads/sites/6/2015/07/20140539/Social-Media-Site-Usage-2014-_-Pew-Research-Centers-Internet-American-Life-Project.pdf

Field, M. J. (1996). *Telemedicine: A guide to assessing telecommunications in health care.* National Academy Press.

Gilbertson, J. (2020). *Telemental health: The essential guide to providing successful online therapy.* PESI.

Gloria, A. M., & Uttal, L. (2020). Conceptual considerations in moving from face-to-face to online teaching. *International Journal on E-Learning, 19*(2), 139–159.

Gonzalez, M. L. S., McCord, C. E., Dopp, A. R., Tarlow, K. R., Dickey, N. J., McMaughan, D. K., & Elliott, T. R. (2019). Telemental health training and delivery in primary care: A case report of interdisciplinary treatment. *Journal of Clinical Psychology, 75*(2), 260–270. https://doi.org/10.1002/jclp.22719

Harrison, K. L. (2021). A call to action: Online learning and distance education in the training of couple and family therapists. *Journal of Marital & Family Therapy, 47*(2), 408–423. https://doi.org/10.1111/jmft.12512

Health Resources and Services Administration. (n.d.). *What is telehealth?* U.S. Department of Health and Human Services. https://telehealth.hhs.gov/patients/understanding-telehealth/

Hjelm, N. M. (2005). Benefits and drawbacks of telemedicine. *Journal of Telemedicine and Telecare, 11*, 60–70. https://doi.org/10.1258/1357633053499886

Howard, A., Flanagan, M., Drouin, M., Carpenter, M., Chen, E., Duchovic, C., & Toscos, T. (2018). Adult experts' perceptions of telemental health for youth: A Delphi study. *JAMIA Open, 1*(1), 67–74.

Hornblow, A. R. (1986). The evolution and effectiveness of telephone counseling services. *Hospital and Community Psychiatry, 37*, 731–733. https://doi.org/10.1176/ps.37.7.731

Kaiser Family Foundation. (2018). *Mental health care health professional shortage areas (HPSAs)*. https://www.kff.org/other/state-indicator/mental-health-care-health-professional-shortage-areas-hpsas

Koukaras, P., Tjortjis, C., & Rousidis, D. (2020). Social media types: Introducing a data driven taxonomy. *Computing, 102*(1), 295–340. https://doi.org/10.1007/s00607-019-00739-y

Lin, J. (2010). Popularity, funding for health-effect research and cell-phone addiction. *Telecommunications Health and Safety, 52*, 164–166.

Merriam-Webster. (n.d.). *Demand*. https://www.merriam-webster.com/dictionary/demand

Moorhouse, B. (2020). Adaptations to a face-to-face initial teacher education course "forced" online due to the COVID-19 pandemic. *Journal of Education for Teaching, 46*(4), 609–611. https://doi.org/10.1080/02607476.2020.1755205

Nesbit, T. (2012). *The role of telehealth in an evolving health care environment: Workshop summary.* National Academies Press.

Orr, D., Weller, M., & Farrow, R. (2018). *Models for online, open, flexible and technology enhanced higher education across the globe—A comparative analysis.* International Council for Distance Education. https://oofat.oerhub.net/OOFAT/

Pew Research Center. (2021, April 7). *Mobile fact sheet.* https://www.pewresearch.org/internet/fact-sheet/mobile/

Ranger, S. (2022, February 25). *What is cloud computing? Everything you need to know about the cloud explained.* ZDNet. https://www.zdnet.com/article/what-is-cloud-computing-everything-you-need-to-know-about-the-cloud/

Rispoli, M., & Machalicek, W. (2020). Advances in telehealth and behavioral assessment and intervention in education: Introduction to the special issue. *Journal of Behavioral Education, 29*, 189–194. https://doi.org/10.1007/s10864-020-09383-5

Siedner, M. J., Harling, G., Reynolds, Z., Gilbert, R. F., Venkataramani, A., & Tsai, A. C. (2020). *Social distancing to slow the US COVID-19 epidemic: An interrupted time-series analysis.* medRxiv.

Snow, W. H., & Coker, K. (2020). Distance counselor education: Past, present, future. *The Professional Counselor, 10*(1), 40–56.

Sommers-Flanagan, J., & Sommers-Flanagan, R. (2017). *Clinical interviewing* (6th ed). Wiley.

Statista. (2022, July 29). *U.S. cost of living: Statistics and facts.* https://www.statista.com/topics/768/cost-of-living/

U.S. Department of Veterans Affairs. (2018, February). *Fact sheet: Telemental health in the Department of Veterans Affairs.* https://www.va.gov/anywheretoanywhere/docs/TeleMental_Health_fact-sheet.PDF

Usher-Pines, L., Raja, P, Quereshi, N., Huskamp, H, Busch, A., & Mehrotra, A. (May 2020). Use of tele-mental health in conjunction with in-person care: A qualitative exploration of implementation models. *Psychiatric Services, 71*(5), 419–426.

Von Hafften, A. (n.d.). *History of telepsychiatry.* American Psychiatric Association. https://www.psychiatry.org/psychiatrists/practice/telepsychiatry/toolkit/history-of-telepsychiatry

World Health Organization. (n.d.). *Mental health.* https://www.who.int/health-topics/mental-health#tab=tab_1

World Health Organization. (2010). *Telemedicine: Opportunities and developments in member states: Report on the second global survey on eHealth.* Author.

Yu, R. P., Ellison, N. B., & Lampe, C. (2018). Facebook use and its role in shaping access to social benefits among older adults. *Journal of Broadcasting & Electronic Media, 62*(1), 71–90. https://doi.org/10.1080/08838151.2017.1402905

Credits

CHAPTER 2

Ethical and Legal Considerations in Telemental Health

Amie A. Manis and Marilyn Montgomery

> Ethics and equity and the principles of justice do not change with the endeavour.
>
> *–D. H. Lawrence*

Learning Objectives

After reading this chapter, you should be able to do the following:

- Identify the relevant codes of ethics and specific code sections to guide your practice of telemental health
- Review federal and state laws governing telemental health counseling and supervision practice relevant to your practice location
- Apply an ethical decision-making model to navigate ethical dilemmas in telemental health

Introduction

Counselors and therapists preparing to enter the field will set foot on territory that is relatively new for the helping professions. Prior to the pandemic that emerged in 2020, ethics training focused primarily on the application of ethical standards in a physical setting. Telemedicine was becoming more common across disciplines but was typically available only to select populations and geographic regions. The massive improvisation that took place to serve those in desperate need of care during the pandemic changed the practice landscape forever, with many expecting some of these changes to be permanent. Providing services via virtual platforms presents new demands for counselors and therapists and brings new ethical challenges—or new twists on familiar ethical challenges—to which professionals must respond.

Developing competence with distance counseling and supervision is not only a 21st-century necessity; it is an ethical responsibility. This is true whether distance services will be at the center of your practice or an approach you adopt to accommodate some clients regularly (e.g., clients with limited mobility or transportation) or occasionally (e.g., inclement weather). Recently, advocacy for the counseling profession and the clients it serves is yielding positive results as a number of states have introduced and enacted interstate counseling compact legislation to allow licensed professional counselors residing in compact member states to practice in other compact member states without the need for multiple licenses (National Center for Interstate Compacts, 2022). This is increasingly feasible through distance platforms and may significantly broaden your reach to populations you wish to serve. Chapter 1 provided important historical context for advances in telemental health and introduced information you will need to know as you consider how to integrate technology into your training and practice. Our aim in this chapter is to provide you with the information and tools you will need to align your practice of telemental health with current and relevant professional ethical codes as well as applicable international, federal, and state laws.

More than ever before, being nimble and adapting to change will be essential throughout your career. Technological changes that allow people to interact in heretofore unimagined ways will continue to evolve. Professional ethics and laws, however, will evolve more slowly in response to new issues and opportunities that arise. While new technological platforms seem to appear overnight, professional codes of ethics are revised and updated on a cyclical basis by panels of experts in the field; this takes time, discussion, and deliberation. Federal and state laws and rules governing telehealth were adapted as the delivery of health care at a distance became a necessity in early 2020. These continue to expand via amendments and the introduction of new legislation, like the Counseling Compact, to address societal changes and leverage new technologies in making mental health care more accessible. Nevertheless, there will always be instances where you cannot locate a law or rule to dictate your best practice in a tricky situation. Instead, you'll need to rely on ethical codes and the more general guidance they provide, as well as your critical decision-making skills, to decide how to handle ethical dilemmas that may not be specifically legislated. As always, while you are in training you will work closely with your clinical supervisor to mentor you as you navigate this territory.

Living Out an Ethical Commitment

Professional codes of ethics are fundamental in many ways. They bind us together with a set of shared values that guides our practice and, in essence, forms the fiber of our professional identity. This is well captured in the preamble to the current American Counseling Association's (ACA) 2014 code of ethics: "Professional values are an important way of living out an ethical commitment" (p. 3). As this statement implies, a commitment to being ethical is embodied in chosen values; our values, in turn, give us guidance for deciding on the best courses of action within the scope of our profession. As D. H. Lawrence suggested in the quote that begins this chapter, ethics and the values they embody are enduring. They don't shift to fit the circumstances (or practice population, modality, or setting). Instead, they are a steadfast lighthouse to guide your way and navigate practice decisions safely.

We imagine this concept resonates with you as someone who has chosen to enter a helping profession. If you have already completed a course in counseling ethics you have discovered that your training is preparing you to go much deeper than simply knowing the ethical codes. You are becoming a member of a profession. Becoming a professional counselor or therapist involves a process of internalizing an identity that embodies a shared ethical commitment to the public. Through the integration and development that takes place as you engage with your classmates, professors, supervisors, and mentors, you are developing a "therapeutic self" that "combines the professional (roles, decisions, ethics) and personal (values, morals, perception)…and provides a frame of reference for ethical practice" (Lloyd-Hazlett & Foster, 2017, p. 91).

Students, educators, and licensed practitioners are all bound by the code of ethics set by their profession. These are articulated by professional associations (e.g., the ACA) and credentialing and licensing bodies. For example, organizations like the Center for Credentialing & Education (CCE, n.d.), introduced in Chapter 1, offer a number of credentials with specific codes of ethics, including one for telemental health providers: Board Certified Telemental Health Provider (BC-TMH). In addition, the ACA (2022) has recently published information on state licensing boards that require licensed professional counselors to adhere to the ACA 2014 code of ethics. As you acquire a license and/or credential in your field of practice and establish professional memberships, you will need to align your practice to each respective code of ethics. For example, a licensed professional counselor who is a member of ACA and credentialed as an approved clinical supervisor (ACS) by CCE is required to align their practice with both the current ACA code of ethics and the ACS code of ethics (CCE, 2008).

You might be wondering how you will keep up with all of the codes and laws that will apply to you. Fortunately, there is significant similarity and overlap in the ethical codes of the mental health professions, and there are similarities between the codes and with the laws regulating the practice of mental health services. Where there are gaps or disagreements, the rule of thumb is to practice to the highest ethical standard that applies to your license and profession. Similarly, if you are working through an ethical decision-making model to resolve a dilemma, you should consult all relevant codes and construct a response that upholds the highest standard.

TIME TO BOOKMARK!

ACA's Knowledge Center: State-by-state licensure requirements	https://www.counseling.org/knowledge-center/licensure-requirements
National Center for Interstate Compacts: FAQ for Counselors	https://counselingcompact.org/faq/

As you recall, the aim of this chapter is to help you grow your familiarity with ethical and legal considerations in telemental health. Another aim is to help you identify the most current and relevant code(s) of ethics and laws for your own field of practice and location. Review the links in Table 2.1 for the most recent ethical codes available for the profession (or professions) for which you are preparing and any credentials you already hold or plan to seek (e.g., certified substance abuse counselor [CSAC] or national certified counselor [NCC]) and look for the standards that have relevance to telemental health.

Additionally, look at the ethical codes for professions with whom you are likely to collaborate, as individuals from several helping professionals often interact to provide clients with care (e.g., school counselors and school social workers). What similarities and differences do you see in the ethical guidelines pertaining to distance client care across helping professions?

TABLE 2.1   **Counseling and Related Professional Codes of Ethics**

American Association of Marriage and Family Therapists (AAMFT)   *2015 Code of Ethics*   https://www.aamft.org/Legal_Ethics/Code_of_Ethics.aspx
American Counseling Association (ACA)   *2014 Code of Ethics*   https://www.counseling.org/resources/aca-code-of-ethics.pdf
American Mental Health Counselors Association (AMHCA)   *2020 Code of Ethics*   https://www.amhca.org/HigherLogic/System/DownloadDocumentFile.ashx?DocumentFileKey=24a27502-196e-b763-ff57-490a12f7edb1
American School Counselor Association (ASCA)   *2016 Ethical Standards for School Counselors*   https://www.schoolcounselor.org/About-School-Counseling/Ethical-Legal-Responsibilities/ASCA-Ethical-Standards-for-School-Counselors-(1)

American Psychological Association (APA) *2017 Ethical Principles of Psychologists and Code of Conduct* https://www.apa.org/ethics/code/ethics-code-2017.pdf
Center for Credentialing *Access Ethics by Credential (e.g., Board Certified Telemental Health Provider; BC-TMH)* https://www.cce-global.org/credentialing/ethics/acs
Commission on Rehabilitation Counselor Certification *2017 Code of Ethics for Certified Rehabilitation Counselors* https://crccertification.com/wp-content/uploads/2021/03/CRC_CodeEthics_Eff2017-Final_newdiesign.pdf
NAADAC, The Association for Addiction Professionals *2021 Code of Ethics* https://www.naadac.org/code-of-ethics
National Career Development Association (NCDA) *2015 Code of Ethics* https://www.ncda.org/aws/NCDA/asset_manager/get_file/3395
National Association of Social Workers (NASW) *2021 Code of Ethics* https://www.socialworkers.org/About/Ethics/Code-of-Ethics/Code-of-Ethics-English
National Board for Certified Counselors *2016 Code of Ethics* https://www.nbcc.org/assets/Ethics/NBCCCodeofEthics.pdf

Formalized codes of ethics have been developed for nearly every profession, embodying the values, ideals, and guiding principles for action they seek to uphold. As you likely

VOICES FROM THE FIELD

How have you met the challenge of continuing care (ethically and legally) for clients who relocate?

"Right now I am licensed in two states after a client moved across state lines and wanted to continue therapy with me. I was able to obtain full clinical licensure through the second state's relatively easy forms and application process. As counselors we abide by a code of ethics, and these ethical values translate across state lines. I carefully reviewed the laws in the second state, and there were no specific differences. In the case of mandated reporting, I would contact the respective states' authorities for both children and family services or emergency services if confidentiality needed to be broken. If ever there is another client that would like to continue, I will assess the laws and regulations of the respective state and continue to obtain licensure!"

–Jennifer Bonino, PhD, LCPC, NCC, Chicago, IL

noticed, all ethical codes have a similar "look and feel," but there are also differences in content and emphasis.

It would be burdensome to walk through all of the codes of ethics that apply to mental health professionals working in distance settings in this chapter. So, in the next section, we dive deeply into the ethical code for professional counselors, particularly the sections that are relevant to the provision of telemental health in a digital age. This will provide you with an example of how one profession has taken on the challenge of providing guidance for the ethical practice of distance services.

2014 ACA Code of Ethics

The ACA is considered a professional home for all counselors. As such, we want to draw your attention to the codes that comprise Section H of the 2014 ACA code of ethics. This section articulates standards related to distance counseling and the use of technology in counseling and social media; this was an important addition in the last update to the code.

At the time the updated code of ethics was released, Meyers (2014) provided an overview of the process that occurs about every 10 years, and in this case involved substantive additions and updates to the 2005 ACA code of ethics. She quoted the task force chair, Perry Francis, to capture the nature of a code of ethics as a "living document that is meant to change as the profession grows and develops over time" (para. 4). The 11 members of the ACA Ethics Revision Task Force recognized the changing nature of society and its impact on counseling practice since the 2005 code of ethics was issued, creating new guidelines in Section H. Yet no one could have imagined the emergent need for this guidance when the global pandemic of 2020 resulted in widespread telehealth practice across the helping professions and created the need for additional clarity about ethical practice in an evolving society.

Section H: Distance Counseling, Technology, and Social Media

While it may seem obvious, delivering counseling at a distance doesn't change any of the fundamentals of ethical practice, only how they translate in a new setting (Barnett & Kolmes, 2016). For example, while counselors remain accountable to the entire 2014 ACA code of ethics, Section H calls for our *active* engagement in keeping up with the evolution of practice with respect to distance counseling, technology, and social media. It requires us to make every effort to practice knowledgably, especially when it comes to protecting client confidentiality and aligning our use of technology to legal and ethical provisions. It specifically addresses six major areas of practice:

- Knowledge and legal considerations
- Informed consent and security
- Client verification

- Distance counseling relationship
- Records and web maintenance
- Social media

These encompass a total of 21 standards. In this section, we draw your attention to the obligations of professional counseling students and practitioners in each of the six areas, with an emphasis on examples drawn from the field.

Section H.1: Knowledge and Legal Considerations

Section H.1 consists of two codes that articulate the responsibility to develop the knowledge and skills necessary for distance counseling, the use of technology, and/or the use of social media. One specific knowledge base which, as you know, is evolving, relates to working with clients in other states or countries. Since these standards are broad in addressing the use of technology in counseling as well as social media, they hold relevance for all professional counselors.

Knowledge and Competency

Section H.1.a requires counselors to develop the knowledge and skills necessary for effective distance counseling, use of technology, and/or social media. These encompass technical, ethical, and legal domains. Chapter 1 of this book provided you with an overview of resources for training in telemental health, which you may want to refer back to as you plan your own professional development. We also encourage you to explore options within your department, university, and local and state associations for training. Opportunities for training burgeoned during the pandemic-related expansion of telemental health and continue to increase; those entering the profession see the need to become informed, particularly with respect to distance counseling ethics and laws (Johnson & Rehfuss, 2021).

Laws and Statutes

Section H.1.b addresses a counselor's responsibility to know the laws and regulations to be followed based on their own location *and* the client's location. In addition, counselors hold a responsibility to make themselves and their clients aware of legal rights and limitations related to counseling practice across state lines or international borders. This happens more often than you might think. For example, you may be in a geographic area of the country that borders closely on another state with the opportunity to make counseling available in two states. If license reciprocity has not been established, you may need to be licensed in both states. Or, while you may not intend to see clients beyond your own state, you may have clients who wish to continue services with you after relocating, who leave for college in another state, or who travel for work or pleasure to other states or countries. In those cases, aligning your practice to laws in both locations is required. Later in the chapter we will provide more information and resources to support you in identifying and becoming familiar with the laws in your state and others in which you may wish to practice.

Section H.2: Informed Consent and Security

As with any counseling relationship, clients have the right to make an informed decision about whether to engage with us. On a fundamental level this is no different when the location of counseling is at a distance, technology is employed, or communication occurs on social media. Yet, the introduction of technology does lead to unique ethical considerations related to informed consent and security.

Informed Consent and Disclosure

Section H.2.a introduces specific guidelines for ensuring that clients are fully informed before consenting to distance counseling and/or the use of technology and social media. We would note that while children are not in a position to give informed consent, the practice of establishing assent is one we recommend. Since it has been shown that therapeutic rapport is central to effective counseling, providing developmentally accessible information about the counseling process and relationship is key (Coffman & Barnett, 2021).

There are nine points to be addressed with clients as part of establishing informed consent for counseling at a distance and/or the use of technology and social media. Informed consent is discussed in detail in Chapter 4; for now consider how important it is to inform potential clients of the associated risks and benefits when we integrate technology in counseling. Also, notice how informed consents guide us to prepare clients for the nuts and bolts of the process when we integrate technology with mental health care: (a) distance counseling credentials, physical location of practice, and contact information; (b) risks and benefits of engaging in the use of distance counseling, technology, and/or social media; (c) the possibility of technology failure and alternate methods of service delivery; (d) anticipated response time; (e) emergency procedures to follow when the counselor is not available; (f) time zone differences; (g) cultural and/or language differences that may affect delivery of services; and (h) possible denial of insurance benefits.

TIME TO BOOKMARK!	
Telebehavioral Health Institute: Informed Consent Library	https://www.naadac.org/assets/2416/marlene_maheu_ac17ho2.pdf

Confidentiality Maintained by the Counselor

Section H.2.b requires counselors to inform clients of limits to maintaining the confidentiality of electronic records and/or transmissions. Clients need to be made aware of who may gain authorized or unauthorized access to these records. Examples cited in the code include employees, colleagues, supervisors, and information technology staff or specialists.

Acknowledgement of Limitations

Section H.2.c builds on and reinforces Section H.2.b, stipulating that clients must be informed of the "inherent limitations of confidentiality when using technology." It is our responsibility to ensure that clients are aware that while we take every precaution to safeguard information shared in the counseling process, there are technology related risks when making authorized disclosures. In addition, unauthorized access is a possible risk of which clients need to be aware.

Security

Section H.2.d requires counselors to ensure their websites and technology-based communications are encrypted. Further, the encryption must align with current standards and legal requirements of your practice area. We further address this topic in the section on legal considerations and the responsibility of counselors and their business partners to protect the confidentiality of electronic records at all times, including during authorized transmissions.

Section H.3: Client Verification

Since technology allows us to engage with clients through means such as videoconferencing, telephone, chat, email, or social media platforms, it is important that we establish a process for verifying their identity. Section H.3 specifies that counselors must ensure steps are in place to verify a client's identity not only at the beginning, but throughout the therapeutic process. Examples are offered in the standard, such as a code word, an assigned number, or an image. When counseling at a distance through a HIPAA-compliant videoconferencing platform, some counselors have clients show a driver's license or other photo identification at the beginning of the session. More formal verification like this may be especially important for the intake session with a new client for whom the counselor has no prior visual reference.

Section H.4: The Distance Counseling Relationship

Section H.4 includes six standards that address the distance counseling relationship. These describe our responsibility to inform clients about counseling relationships at a distance, assess their suitability for each client, and provide alternatives if a live, face-to-face format is best for the client. While there is evidence of the effectiveness of telemental health, it may not be an appropriate means of service delivery for everyone (Schaffer et al., 2020).

Benefits and Limitations

Section H.4.a highlights the responsibility of counselors to inform clients about the *benefits and limitations* of using whatever technologies are being used, including but not limited to computer hardware and software, phones, audio and video applications, and storage devices.

Consider online assessments, for example. During the COVID-19 pandemic, school-based career counselors guided students through informed consent related to distance counseling. In addition, they needed to discuss the benefits and limitations of the *web-based* career assessments they used. In some cases, counselors asked their clients to engage in web-based assessments as homework outside of session, then walk through the results while sharing a screen during a session. In other cases, counselors guided clients through an assessment online via a shared screen. In either case, reviewing the benefits and limitations of the technologies being used was required, in addition to explaining the nature and purpose of the assessment and how the results would be used, just as it is when we use technologies in our offices with clients (see ACA, 2014, E.3.a., Explanation to Clients).

Professional Boundaries in Distance Counseling

Establishing and maintaining a professional presence and clear boundaries with clients is central to Section H, and a particular focus of Section H.4.b. Boundary setting in telemental health has been a topic of consideration for some time. Drum and Littleton (2014) suggested best practices in telepsychology, which we summarized in Table 2.2. Notice how these best practices tie to specific sections of the ethical code that will guide your practice. These may also serve to reinforce a fundamental principle of Section H of the 2014 ACA code of ethics: Professional presence and engagement online call for more formality and clearly articulated ground rules and boundaries. This form of communication is distinctly different from the less formal and more relaxed personal presence and engagement to which you may be accustomed.

TABLE 2.2   **Setting Professional Boundaries in Telemental Health**

Best Practice Recommendations	Tips and Strategies
Maintain professional hours and respect timing of sessions	<ul><li>Deliver asynchronous feedback during business hours</li><li>Consider cultural differences when addressing client punctuality</li></ul>
Ensure timely and consistent feedback and manage excessive communications	<ul><li>Inform clients of expected turnaround time at beginning of treatment</li><li>Model appropriate frequency and communications</li></ul>

Ensure a private, consistent, professional and culturally sensitive setting	• Guide clients in taking steps to ensure a private and distraction-free environment for sessions • Explore technology-compliant text-based communications as an alternative if a client's privacy is breached in their location • Be consistent in your location and intentional about establishing a professional and culturally sensitive backdrop on camera • Take steps to prevent background noise and/or use a white noise machine • Dress professionally
Ensure privacy of nonclients	• Guide clients to take steps to ensure the privacy of others in their environment (e.g., keeping photos out of the camera lens; maintaining private space for sessions on camera)
Ensure that the telecommunications used convey professionalism	• Use professional photos and language on websites • Provide visibility and/or links to your professional credentials, associations, and code(s) of ethics • Consider the professionalism of all your online activities • Develop your social media/communication policy and review with clients to ensure their understanding
Model appropriate self-boundaries	• Be intentional about your own wellness • Avoid checking asynchronous communications outside of work • Provide advance notice of leave times and remind clients of emergency procedures
Ensure privacy of the therapist's work	• Establish policies on recording and client access to video and audio communications and safeguard telecommunication files by disabling downloading • Consider setting policy regarding client use and misuse of feedback for inclusion in your informed consent document and process
Use professional language and consider alternative interpretations	• Before sending written communications to clients, review them for clarity and professional tone • Avoid text shorthand, excessive punctuation, and emoticons
Ensure competence in the practice of telepsychology	• Acquire the skills and knowledge you need to confidently apply the technologies you will use • Seek training and consultation within and beyond the field (e.g., web designers and information technology professionals) • Engage in training and continuing education on telemental health and managing a professional online presence

Note: Adapted from "Therapeutic Boundaries in Telepsychology: Unique Issues and Best Practice Recommendations" by K. B. Drum & H. L. Littleton, 2014, *Professional Psychology: Research and Practice, 45*(5), 309–315.

Technology-Assisted Services

Clients must be the first consideration when we decide to engage in distance counseling or integrate technology and/or social media into our practice. Section H.4.c requires us to assess the suitability of applications for our clients. We need to consider a client's intellectual, emotional, physical, linguistic, and functional capacity with respect to the application. In addition, we need to ask ourselves if the application is suitable to meet the client's needs. Further, we must be sure our clients understand why we are using a technology application, and to monitor their use and step in as needed to guide or correct them.

Effectiveness of Services

Similar to the responsibilities outlined in Section H.4.c, we are also charged with monitoring the effectiveness of distance counseling services. If we determine that distant counseling is not effective, we must consider face-to-face services if possible (either offer in-person sessions or, if that is not possible, referral to another provider who offers in-person services).

Access

Section H.4.e addresses the requirement to provide clients with information about *reasonable* access to applications to be used when we provide technology-mediated services. We want to draw your attention to the word *reasonable* as it connects to the assessment of the suitability of technology-assisted services for clients. What is reasonable access for one client may not be reasonable for another.

For instance, while working with counselors in Alaska and other rural areas of the United States and Canada, we learned that clients' access to hardware and reliable and stable internet connections can be limited due to geography and weather. While computer or internet access may be available through a local clinic or school, arranging for technical support and privacy at that site (if indeed a secure platform is available for communications) would be an additional responsibility for the provider.

Another consideration when integrating technology is the cost of applications. Consider the earlier example of utilizing assessments and web resources online in career counseling. In addition to assessing a client's access to an electronic device capable of an internet connection and the availability of internet, we must be cognizant of the costs of applications or assessments as we select and explore the possibility with clients.

Communication Differences in Electronic Media

As noted in section H.4.f, counselors are held accountable for considering the differences between face-to-face and electronic communication and how those may impact the counseling process. Further, it places responsibility on counselors to educate our clients on how to prevent and, when indicated, address misunderstandings that could arise from a lack of audio and/or visual cues (e.g., when using phone calls, email, or chat). How, specifically, will you ensure your clients understand the difference between traditional (face-to-face) and virtual therapy? Will you include material with your informed consent, like a brochure about your practice or links to websites available to the public as a way to leverage technology (Stoll et al., 2020)?

Whatever you decide to use to inform, assess, and prepare your clients for navigating distance counseling, the use of technology, and/or social media, keep in mind that informed consent is much more than walking clients through intake paperwork. Diligence in explaining and ensuring individuals seeking care with us understand and agree to the ground rules for the counseling relationship, process, and format is central to living out our ethical commitment. Consider the potential utility of these websites designed to help the public make an informed decision about engaging in telemental health.

TIME TO BOOKMARK!

Before You Press Record	https://www.camft.org/Resources/Legal-Articles/Chronological-Article-List/before-you-press-record
Is it OK to Record Your Therapy Session?	https://www.huffpost.com/entry/record-therapy-sessions-ok_l_5f6a13c5c5b6968b276fb61f
Virtual Therapy v. In-Person Therapy	https://www.psychology.org/resources/virtual-therapy-vs-in-person/
What You Need to Know Before Choosing Online Therapy	https://www.apa.org/topics/telehealth/online-therapy

Section H.5: Records and Web Maintenance

Section H.5 contains four sections. It begins by building on Section H.2, which you will recall addresses informed consent and security. While these standards also specify the type of information that must be available to our clients, they go further in addressing the maintenance and accessibility of electronic material (e.g., a practice website).

Records

Section H.5.a reinforces the requirement that counselors follow the law in maintaining electronic records. It also introduces our duty to inform clients on how their records are encrypted and secured, and if or for how long they may be archived. This standard underscores the importance of making your own informed decision about a

HIPAA-compliant practice platform and being familiar with its features and security measures. As you move forward in the chapter, you will learn more about the laws that govern electronic record keeping and the shared responsibility health care providers hold with their business partners in safeguarding electronic health records.

Client Rights

Counselors are required to represent our professional credentials accurately as a matter of ethical practice (ACA, 2014). The ACA (n.d.) reminds us that this must include temporary and/or emergency authorizations to practice such as those issued during the pandemic that may have permitted interstate practice or allowed students to expand their scope of practice. Section H.5.b expands attention to conveying such information to the public by stipulating the requirement to provide electronic links to relevant licensing and certification boards to clients. Since these bodies are in place to protect the public, it is important that clients have access to them in the event that ethical concerns or complaints arise.

Electronic Links

Wherever you choose to make electronic links available to your clients, Section H.5.c calls upon us to ensure they are professional in nature, up to date, and working. Consider a strategy for web or other maintenance on a regular cycle, including who will be responsible for your web maintenance. Will it be you, an employee, a firm you contract with to build and maintain your site, or a feature of the telemental health platform you choose? A simple Google search confirms that the World Wide Web is rich in firms advertising website development, reviews of such companies, and key considerations if or when you may decide to develop a professional counseling website.

Multicultural and Disability Considerations

Section H.5.d delves into the accessibility of websites. Of course, the accessibility of the information is important in all aspects of your practice, whether in person, virtual, or a combination of both. The standard also requires us to provide translation capabilities for clients with a different primary language, when feasible. For both, we are required to acknowledge the limitations of the measures we have taken. No doubt you have experienced closed-captioning errors in Zoom or viewed a Zoom transcript with imperfections in translating the spoken word to writing.

You may be wondering what an accessible website looks like, or what goes into ensuring accessibility. The National Center on Disability Access and Access to Education (NCDAE, 2022) has outlined 10 principles of accessible design. These include considerations like formatting to promote readability, including captions for media, ease of navigation, and ensuring the functionality and clarity of links. The World Wide Web Consortium (W3C, 2022) is another organization focused on promoting accessibility as an important aspect of its commitment to seeing the web reach its full potential.

TIME TO GET ONLINE!

Visit the NCDAE (https://ncdae.org/resources/factsheets/principles.php) and W3C (https://www.w3.org/WAI/) websites. Then locate the websites of one or two mental health professionals in your area.

- How well do websites align to the NCDAE's 10 principles?
- Would you find the website easy to use and appealing if you were looking for mental health care?
- Were you able to identify their credentials and the code(s) of ethics they follow?
- If they asked for your review what strengths and opportunities would you note?

Section H.6. Social Media

Since technology has become part of the cultural fabric of the 21st century, it's likely that you are a digital native (or a digital immigrant—yes, that's the term!) and arrived at graduate school with a personal social media presence. According to Meyers (2018), social media platforms like TikTok, YouTube, Facebook, Instagram, and Snapchat are a mainstay of socialization among people of all ages, and for young adults they are central to forming relationships and staying informed. In addition, counselors are increasingly using social media platforms for mental health education and advocacy, to humanize the field, to increase access to mental health resources, and to market their practices (Phillips, 2022).

In 2018, Meyers gathered perspectives from ACA members in a call to counselors to recognize digital presence and communication as an important cultural consideration in counseling. Organizing the strategies proposed in her article in terms of a multicultural counseling and social justice framework (i.e., awareness, knowledge, skill, and action) may help you map out areas of opportunity for professional development (Ratts et al., 2016). First, build awareness through a self-assessment of your own views of social media and an appreciation of its significance in the lives of our clients. Second, develop your knowledge of the benefits and limitations of social media for clients and in practice and share that with clients as part of informed consent. Third, prepare to support clients in making informed decisions about engagement on social media platforms with specific consideration of safety and mental health. And fourth, evaluate opportunities to use social media as a platform for mental health education and advocacy.

Section H.6 of the 2016 ACA code of ethics is in place to guide counselors on the intersection of social media with counseling practice. This section addresses managing a professional virtual presence, addressing social media in the informed consent process, client privacy with respect to their social media presence, and maintaining confidentiality on public social media. This section of the code may apply to counselors with an online presence, regardless of whether they engage in distance counseling. If you plan to be a counselor with a website advertising an in-person practice this section will apply to you!

"Virtual Professional Presence" (H.6.a) is the focus of the first of the four standards. It stipulates that if a counselor wishes to use social media it is essential to ensure the separation of personal and professional social media presence. One step we recommend for graduate students is to evaluate and carefully moderate your personal presence on social media and review who has access. Consider what your personal profiles, posts, photos, or videos may be communicating to the public. For example, imagine the impact of a seemingly benign social media post where you are enjoying happy hour on vacation or gathered with friends for a drink after work and put yourself in the mind-set of an adolescent client struggling with substance use.

Deciding if or how you will establish a professional presence on social media merits careful thought and planning. Consider these tips from Phillips (2022):

- Grab people's attention.
- Don't compare yourself to others.
- Develop a thick skin.
- Find support.
- Remember, it's hard work!

In addition to these tips, Phillips highlighted the creative strategies of several counselors with a professional social media presence to humanize the field, educate and advocate, and market their practices. These include posting short videos, generating educational content based on user questions about mental health, and using limited self-disclosure to normalize the experience of mental health concerns and help seeking, and provide links to resources.

"Social Media as Part of Informed Consent" (H.6.b) is the second standard. It requires that counselors inform clients of the benefits and limitations of social media. Further, communicating boundaries for the use of social media within the counseling relationship is a critical aspect of ethical practice. For example, Phillips (2022) interviewed counselors who utilize social media platforms to educate, advocate, and/or market their practices, and the interviews reinforced the importance of setting and communicating clear guidelines for engagement. This could include informing clients your presence on social media may be limited to posting information. Further, if we are using social media as a tool to educate, consider using a social media content disclaimer distinguishing education from therapy. Providing links to resources for locating a mental health provider and additional resources may help clarify and address limitations.

Client Virtual Presence

Section H.6.c requires that we respect our clients' privacy on social media. Similar to explaining the limits of our own social media engagement, it is also important that clients understand we will respect their boundaries. Therefore, we want clients to be aware that we will only view their social media with their consent—or not all. In addition to preserving client privacy, it also limits any expectation that we may be monitoring social media in a way that infers we would be aware of crises, or in worst-case scenarios, threats of harm to self or others.

TIME TO GET ONLINE!

Locate and review a few therapists' websites and social media pages.

- Do they include client testimonials? If they do, how is the client's identity protected?
- Do you see clear differentiation of personal and professional roles?
- Is education or advocacy about telemental health provided?
- Identify and discuss practices you see that uphold ethical guidelines on telemental health practice and some that seem questionable or even unethical (or potentially illegal).

Use of Public Social Media

Finally, Section H.6.d mandates counselors to take precautions to avoid the public disclosure of confidential information on social media. For example, consider the steps you would need to take to post client testimonials while protecting their identity. Further, just as you would not acknowledge a client while out shopping unless they speak to you, manage any social media engagement within the policies you set with clients so as not to divulge your professional relationship to others.

Legal Considerations and Telemental Health

In addition to aligning your distance counseling practice to the highest ethical standards related to your professional licenses and/or credentials, you must also attend to federal and state laws governing telemental health practices and, if applicable, international laws. At the beginning of the chapter, we emphasized the evolving nature of professional ethics and laws with respect to telehealth practices along with state-specific differences. Advocacy initiatives to facilitate interstate compacts aimed at making telehealth services more accessible have gained traction and momentum since the COVID-19 pandemic began. In addition, pandemic-related emergency orders and exceptions to allow greater flexibility in delivering health care have also contributed to the dynamic nature of legal considerations. It is critical for counselors to be informed about federal and state laws as they stand, and to put tools and strategies in place to remain alert to a rapidly changing legislative landscape. This section of the chapter is designed to support you in just that: preparing for informed telemental health practice within and outside of your state as needed and building resources to remain abreast of legislative updates and changes.

Protected Health Information

The U.S. Department of Health and Human Services (HHS) administers and enforces privacy rules related to health care information in both paper and electronic form. There is little doubt that you are already familiar with the Health Insurance Portability and Accountability Act of 1996 (HIPAA) in a personal and/or professional capacity. What you may not know is that the initial act was intended primarily, as the name suggests, to ensure the portability of health insurance coverage. It was also enacted in an effort to reduce fraud, encourage the use of medical savings accounts, and improve access to long-term care and insurance. Like our professional ethics, HIPAA has continued to adapt and expand with the times.

The HIPAA Privacy Rule

In 2003 the HIPAA Privacy Rule or Title 1 of HIPAA was introduced. According to HHS, which offers a detailed history of the Privacy Rule (highlighted throughout this section), it established national standards for the protection of medical records and identifiable health information in any medium (e.g., records located in a practice office or clinic) and regulation of its disclosure (Office of Civil Rights [OCR], 2021). This is referred to as *protected health information* (PHI). It requires relevant health care professionals (e.g., doctors and counselors) and organizations (e.g., insurance companies), referred to as covered entities, to ensure measures are in place to safeguard PHI. It also confers the right to individuals to examine and request copies of, or corrections to, their health records. Since its enactment in 2003 there have been modifications followed by opportunities for public comment.

The HIPAA Security Rule

In 2005 the HIPAA Security Rule, or Title II of HIPAA, went further by establishing national standards to protect electronic PHI. This expanded the responsibility of covered entities to put technical safeguards in place to allow for electronic PHI availability while preventing improper use or disclosure of PHI. Altogether, with the advent of the HIPAA Security Rule, covered entities must ensure administrative (e.g., policies and procedures), technical (e.g., encryption of electronic PHI), and physical (e.g., electronic permissions to access to data) safeguards are in place.

HITECH Act

The HITECH Act, ratified in 2009, fortified the HIPAA Privacy and Security Rules as part of an initiative to promote the use of health information technology (e.g., electronic health records). It introduced a requirement for covered entities and their business associates (e.g., companies offering HIPAA-compliant telepractice management software such as Doxy.me) to enter a *business associate contract* (BAC), which you may also see referred to as a *business associate agreement* (BAA). These contracts are required to restrict the disclosure of PHI by any business associate(s) of a covered entity in accordance with the HIPAA Security Rule and to require the implementation of administrative, physical, and technical controls to protect PHI. Further, the HITECH Act (a) established requirements for annual guidance to be issued to covered entities and their business associates on appropriate safeguards, (b) increased penalties for HIPAA violations to include both business associates and covered entities, (c) required the investigation of reported breaches by HHS, (d) expanded individual rights to include access to electronic to records in electronic form, (e) required notification of breaches for unencrypted PHI, and (f) broadened the definition of a breach.

HIPAA Breach Notification Rule

The 2009 requirement for notification of security breaches for nonencrypted information under the HITECH Act laid the ground for the HIPAA Breach Notification Rule. This rule requires covered entities to notify individuals impacted by an unauthorized acquisition, use, or disclosure of PHI of the breach in a timely manner (i.e., no later than 60 days following discovery of a breach) if there is a significant risk of harm (e.g., financial or reputational). In the case of a large-scale breaches (i.e., more than 500 people) the covered entities are also required to notify the HHS Office for Civil Rights within the 60-day timeframe, whereas in the case of small breaches covered entities must notify within 60 days of the end of the calendar year in which the breach occurred.

So, what does all of this federal legislation mean for you? As a health care provider you are considered a covered entity. As a covered entity you are required to adhere to HIPAA to protect your clients' PHI by putting administrative (e.g., who has access to paper or electronic health records), technological (e.g., encryption of electronic PHI), and physical (e.g., how your office or computer is secured) controls in place. Further, as you select and utilize technology to deliver counseling you must enter a contract with your business associates, which binds you in safeguarding the PHI of your clients.

State Privacy Protection Laws

In addition to adhering to the federal laws for protecting PHI, it is important to be aware of state privacy laws, as they may vary. Some states may have more stringent laws (e.g., California and New York) or specific laws that regulate the collection and storage of PHI (HHS, 2021). Further, while some states regulate privacy protection by industry, there is momentum toward greater standardization with state enactments of comprehensive privacy bills. The International Association of Privacy Professionals (IAPP) actively tracks the status of state legislation and the movement toward comprehensive laws (Lively, 2022). The Telehealth Certification Institute (TCI, 2022) is also an excellent resource for training and tools to identify state telemental health laws, rules, and regulations by state *and* by specific health professions.

TIME TO BOOKMARK!

AAMFT Coronavirus and State/ Provincial Telehealth Guidelines	https://www.aamft.org/Events/State_Guide_for_Telehealth.aspx
Guide to Privacy and Security of Health Information	https://www.healthit.gov/sites/default/files/pdf/privacy/onc_privacy_and_security_chapter4_v1_022112.pdf
States' Telemental Health Laws, Rules, and Regulations	https://www.telementalhealthtraining.com/states-rules-and-regulations
Telehealth, HHS	https://telehealth.hhs.gov/providers/legal-considerations/
U.S. State Privacy Legislation Tracker	https://iapp.org/resources/article/us-state-privacy-legislation-tracker/

Protecting Yourself: Liability Insurance

In addition to emphasizing the protection of client health information, HHS (2021) also raises liability and malpractice protection under legal considerations for providers offering telehealth services. Whether you plan to practice telemental health within the borders of the state in which you reside or you plan to serve clients in neighboring states, it is critical that you consult with your insurance provider. There may be limits to coverage or additional coverage required.

As a graduate student you will also be required to have liability insurance before engaging in supervised practice during your clinical practicum and/or internship. There may be limits to coverage for telemental health or specific requirements regarding the qualifications of designated supervisors in place (ACA, n.d.). For example, for graduate students insured through HPSO as a student member of ACA, five criteria must be met for coverage of telebehavioral health counseling sessions as a trainee. Use this checklist for your own insurance check-up as you prepare for supervised counseling practice:

Y/N   Does my site supervisor's license permit the practice of telebehavioral health?

Y/N   Is my site supervisor trained to provide both clinical services and supervision for this type of service delivery?

Y/N   Have or am I scheduled to receive proper training to facilitate telebehavioral sessions?

Y/N   Will my site supervisor be available for me or the client, as needed?

Y/N   Has my site supervisor and/or placement site confirmed that the funding sources for each client session allows me to provide counseling?

State Licensure Laws

Counseling is a relatively new profession as compared to psychiatry, social work, and psychology. This helps to account for the variation in state-based regulation of licensure as the adoption of counseling as a licensed profession happened over time, one state at a time. While state boards play an important role in ensuring public safety through the regulation of health professions, lack of a national standard for counselor licensure contributes to challenges in providing care for clients who are temporarily or permanently out of state, as well as accepting clients who live in another state.

Historically, seeking licensure in another state was the primary means available to counselors wishing to serve a client or clients in another state. Despite advocacy for licensure portability on a national level and emergency orders issued by some states during the pandemic, this may still be a need and a reasonable consideration for some counselors. Registration as a volunteer to provide services across state lines may also be an avenue to explore if interstate practice is a possibility you need to explore to provide continuity of care to a client(s).

As you anticipate postgraduate supervised practice and work toward licensure in your state, it's likely you have visited the website for the state board to which you will apply for licensure or certification. It's also likely you have an idea of the detailed nature of the regulations governing the practice of counseling in your state. You may be aware that when it comes to preparing to practice with a client located in another state, if such practice is permitted *you will have to abide by the laws governing practice in both states*. In this section, we guide you through key considerations and suggest sources for information you will need to complete your own research on telemental health practice in and beyond your state of residence.

Any clinician planning to practice telemental health must consult with their state licensing board for current regulations, remain abreast of changes or updates by regularly visiting the board's website (as regulations for telehealth and telemental health practice are exceptionally dynamic,) and document all consultations and guidance received (Barnett & Kolmes, 2016; Reinhardt, 2019). Repeating this step with the board(s) for any other state in which you wish to practice is also a critical step in evaluating if, and under what terms, you may practice across state lines. Another often referenced resource recommended by Reinhardt (2019) is Epstein Becker Green's Telemental Health/Behavioral Survey, now available as a complimentary app to access their "comprehensive compilation of state telehealth laws, regulations, and policies with the mental/behavioral health practice disciplines" (Lerman & Ozinal, 2021, p. 1).

WHAT WENT WRONG HERE?

Consider the following case brought before a state regulatory board against a licensed counselor (LPC) who provided telemental health services through a mental health therapy mobile application (app). For over a year, the LPC used the app to provide services to a recently divorced client. The app-based therapy involved text exchanges to address the client's depression and post-divorce social adjustment. The counselor's remarks to the client included unprofessional language, personal views, and professional boundary transgressions. For example, the counselor declared that trying to help the client was like Groundhog Day, going over and over the same issues again, and suggesting that they were soulmates and should hang out together next time the ex was in town for time with the kids.

Feeling distressed, the client brought the counselor's behavior to the attention of the therapy app. The app administrators reported the counselor to her state board of licensed professional counselors. Upon investigating, the board learned that in addition to the dubious texts, the counselor had not maintained a client health care information record (the only records were the texts stored on the app), had done no assessments, and formulated no counseling goals or progress notes. *Want to guess what happened?*

The board determined that the counselor had violated state and federal statutes and regulations, as well as the ACA's code of ethics, and required the counselor to surrender her license and pay a $1,000 fine (her malpractice insurance paid most of her legal fees). They also reported this disciplinary action to the National Practitioner Data Base (NPDB). The NPDB was established in 1986 by the U.S. Congress to prevent practitioners from moving state to state without disclosing previous malpractice. Additional information about this case is located on the Healthcare Providers Service Organization (HPSO, n.d.) website.

Insurance Coverage for Telemental Health Care

Be aware that insurance coverage of telemental health care is not universal. The ACA recommends contacting each client's insurance provider and collaborating with the client to establish what is needed for accurate billing. Telephone inquiries are specifically recommended, as websites may be out of date. Consider exploring the sites provided or exploring the website(s) of your professional associations to research insurance coverage and advocacy initiatives.

Limitations to Confidentiality

Once you decide to offer telemental health care in another state, whether you are extending care to a single client who is on vacation or accepting clients on a regular basis, you will need to research each state's laws for navigating exceptions to

---

TIME TO BOOKMARK!

ACA's Government Affairs and Public Policy page	https://www.counseling.org/government-affairs/public-policy
ACA's Knowledge Center	https://www.counseling.org/knowledge-center/mental-health-resources/trauma-disaster/telehealth-information-and-counselors-in-health-care/telebehavioral-health-insurance-and-billing
NBCC's Grassroots Action Center	https://www.votervoice.net/NBCCGrassroots/home

---

confidentiality. Section B of the 2014 ACA code of ethics addresses requirements related to serious and foreseeable harm (B.2.a), end-of-life decisions (B.2.c), and contagious, life-threatening diseases (B.2.c). Counselors are directed to consider applicable laws in the language of each of these standards. In practice, this means that we must know the laws related to these phenomena not only in our state, but also in the state(s) in which our clients reside. The National Conference of States Legislatures (NCSL), a bipartisan organization established in 1975, is a credible resource with a mission that encompasses the exchange of information among state legislatures. It provides visibility to state-by-state requirements related to our ethical and legal responsibilities to protect clients at risk of harm to self or others, to report suspected abuse to vulnerable populations (e.g., minors, the elderly, and the differently abled), and to warn individuals in the event of threats of serious violence.

Duty to Warn

Do you remember studying *Tarasoff v. The Regents of the University of California*? This 1976 case led to legislation in most states either requiring or permitting mental health professionals to warn individuals at risk of harm from a client. As you plan for telemental health practice across state borders, it is critically important that you are familiar with the laws in your own state *and* the state(s) in which your clients are located at the time of service. The NCSL provides a national map depicting the states with laws, whether there is a mandatory duty to warn, and if the duty varies by profession. Further, it's possible to search for additional detail by state.

We would like to mention, however, that *knowing* you have a duty to warn in your state (if your client presents a clear and immediate probability of physical harm to themselves, other individuals, or to society) is one thing, and knowing how you would actually go about doing is a different thing. One of us (Marilyn) was once awakened by phone call from a former client seen for marital issues who declared that things weren't working out with his spouse (from whom he was separated), so he was going to shoot himself—this was especially alarming because I knew that children, and weapons, were in the home. Leaving the client's motivations for making this call aside for other discussion, simply figuring out how to reach appropriate law enforcement in the county where the client had relocated took up precious time. Clearly, simply *knowing* that we have a duty to warn is not the end of our ethical responsibility. When providing distance counseling, not only must you be prepared to do an effective suicide assessment and intervention with appropriate documentation and follow-up with the usual best practices, you also must be ready to involve emergency or support services at the client's location (Luxton et al., 2016).

End-of-Life Decisions

While end-of-life decisions may not be a regular consideration in your practice, it is also important to be familiar with the laws in your state and other states in which you may practice. Since a main objective for this chapter is to provide you with resources to conduct your own research, we suggest exploring and bookmarking the State Statute Navigator provided by Death with Dignity, a national leader in advocacy for people with terminal illness. We also recognize that this is a topic that is likely to require deep personal reflection and may call for implementation of an ethical decision-making model in navigating differences in personal and professional value systems. So, in addition to the State Statute Navigator we would also recommend Irvin Yalom's book, *A Matter of Life and Death* (Yalom & Yalom, 2021). I (Amie) had the opportunity to hear Yalom speak at ACA's 2021 conference about his experience writing it with his wife when she developed a terminal illness and ultimately made the decision to end her life with dignity.

Mandated Reporting

Mental health professionals are among the designated professionals legally required to report suspected abuse to vulnerable populations (e.g., minors, elderly, and differently abled). Since laws and processes may differ from state to state, it is important to be familiar with the laws in all states in which you may practice *and* the process of making a report. There are two excellent sources of information for identifying the laws governing mandated reporting in each state. The Child Welfare Information Gateway hosts a State Statutes Search feature.

As members of an aging society in which we recognize the biopsychosocial strain on family caregivers, we must also remain alert for the possibility of elder abuse (National Alliance for Caregiving and the American Association of Retired Persons, 2020). The U.S. Department of Justice provides comprehensive information related to older adults and state statutes, including a link to Adult Protective Services Reporting laws by state, hosted by the American Bar Association's Commission on Law and Aging. These resources will be important if you engage in telemental health care with clients (or the elderly individuals about whom they relay information) who are residing or temporarily located in another state.

Suicide Prevention

Another important consideration with distance practice is suicide prevention. We need to be familiar with resources available to clients at risk of harming themselves, and we need to know the state laws governing when to breach confidentiality. As a college counselor in the years immediately following the mass shooting at Virginia Tech, I (Amie) carefully tracked proposed legislation and adjusted my practice to the change in Virginia laws regarding informing parents of college students who had reached legal maturity. For more information on resources for suicide prevention and access to a state activities tracker visit the Suicide Prevention Resource Center.

As noted with previous instances when counselors may need to breach confidentiality, the situation becomes more complex as clients are in a different state. For example, in another situation involving a suicide threat, my (Marilyn) client phoned from an undisclosed location to convey "[his] last goodbye and thanks" before he connected his trailer to his car exhaust. He had been traveling several weeks around the country in his motor home, during which time we had met by phone for sporadic counseling check-in sessions. He refused to disclose his specific location, and my surreptitious outreach to law enforcement informed me that, at least at that time, the call could not be traced so that help could be dispatched. Fortunately, my training had given me tools to keep this client, and other duty-to-warn clients talking and alive to see another day. Also fortunately, I had peer supervision relationships that supported me in debriefing both alarming incidents. The importance of this practice for sustaining counselor well-being will be discussed later in this chapter.

International Telemental Health Practice

As we live and work in an increasingly global community you may be interested in making telemental health care available to individuals abroad or encounter a need to continue to offer care to a client who travels abroad for work for extended periods. As you may imagine, just as with interstate differences, there are country-by-country regulations that must be researched and evaluated. Bodulovic et al. (2020) introduced the Global Telehealth Comparison website, hosted by the global law firm DLA Piper, to help provide guidance for providing telehealth care across international borders.

TIME TO BOOKMARK!

American Bar Association's Commission on Law and Aging	https://www.americanbar.org/content/dam/aba/administrative/law_aging/2020-elder-abuse-reporting-chart.pdf?eType=EmailBlastContent&eId=ed64ab8e-28fa-405b-930d-f4d812fb840d
Child Welfare Information Gateway State Statutes Search	https://www.childwelfare.gov/topics/systemwide/laws-policies/state/
Death with Dignity State Statute Navigator	https://deathwithdignity.org/resources/state-statute-navigator/
Global Telehealth Comparison	https://www.dlapiperintelligence.com/telehealth
National Conference of States Legislatures	https://www.ncsl.org/
Suicide Prevention State Activities Tracker	https://sprc.org/states
U.S. Department of Justice State Elder Abuse Statutes	https://www.justice.gov/elderjustice/elder-justice-statutes-0

Ethics and Supervision

Learning from experts is a longstanding tradition in the health professions. First, you master the facts, sharpen your critical thinking, and begin taking on a professional identity of a practitioner in your chosen field. Next, you practice applying all that "book learning" to real people in a closely supervised setting. This first happens while you are still in training. It is your school and fieldwork site's responsibility to provide you with supervisors who are knowledgeable and well versed in the best treatment practices and ethical code of your field (Machuca & Kurns, 2021; Wrape & McGinn, 2019).

Once you graduate, you'll almost certainly have another period (usually at least 2 years) where you are working with clients but required to meet regularly with a supervisor who is qualified according to the requirements of the state license you are pursuing. States typically have regulations regarding the provision of post-degree experience hours by a qualified supervisor. We encourage you to find the regulations concerning supervision for licensure in your field on your current state's website.

You probably have a mental picture of what this supervision will look like (and yes, you'll have many hours of it!). You likely guessed that supervision also has ethical guidelines for its practice. Not surprisingly, the 2014 ACA code of ethics offers guidance for online supervision (F.2.c), stating that supervisors must be competent in the use of the technologies they use in supervision and "take necessary precautions to protect the confidentiality of all information transmitted through any electronic means" (p. 13). In addition, a task force was created by the Association of Counselor Educators and Supervisors (ACES, 2011) to delineate guidelines for the practices that support supervisors' work, thus offering ethical and legal protection for supervisors, supervisees, and clients. Not surprisingly, section 7, titled "Ethical Considerations," delineates specifics for ethical supervision, including confidentiality, the infusion of ethical discussions throughout supervision, and the reporting of ethical breaches. In addition, a best practice for conducting supervision (4.i) specifically addresses technology. When technology is used for distance supervision, the supervisor must approximate face-to-face supervision in allowing both parties to attend to nonverbal as well as verbal behavior to "enhance the supervisor process and the development of the supervisee" (p. 6).

Once you are mature in your career, you may seek out training to become one of these qualified supervisors in your practice setting. One option available to licensed counselors is to become an approved clinical supervisor through NBCC. You may remember the example of a licensed professional counselor who also holds an ACS from earlier in the chapter. Anyone holding the ACS credential is required to abide by the ACS program code of ethics. This code also addresses electronic and distance communications in Section C (CCE, 2016). Review your state licensure board to determine the requirements to be an approved supervisor in your state. Also, mentioned earlier in this chapter, once you begin seeing clients, most training programs will require you, as well as your supervisor, to have malpractice insurance. The insurer will almost certainly stipulate that if you are providing telemental health care, your supervisor must also be knowledgeable about processes and best practices of providing distance client care so that they can support and guide you as you do so (Machuca & Kurns, 2021).

We want to point out, though, that your supervisor can only assist you with what you bring to the discussion. If you've made a mistake or sense that you might be stepping into ethical hot water, bring it to your supervisor. Earlier is better than later. Your supervisor will be knowledgeable about prevalent ethical violations and will help you minimize the likelihood of these occurring or will help you set things right if something has occurred—but only if you've been upfront about your concerns. In supervision, there is no such thing as a stupid question (except for the question you didn't ask)!

Professional Responsibility and Your Own Well-Being

As we envision you eagerly taking on the challenge of providing distance services, we know you will be meeting clients' needs in ways that could not have been imagined only a generation ago—and we feel excitement for you! Nevertheless, we have one more thing for you to consider, and that is this: missteps. For instance, when do mistakes in client care happen? When are errors made in documentation? When are counselors and therapists most likely to cross boundary lines and harm clients?

We assert that no student or practitioner gets up in the morning planning to get into ethical or legal hot water. What we have seen much more often is that when students or practitioners suffer from poor ethical judgment, it is because they have neglected the imperative practice of supporting their own well-being. Many ethical codes stipulate that mental health professionals engage in self-care that maintains and promotes "their own emotional, physical, mental, and spiritual wellbeing." And why must this be done? It's so they can "best meet their professional responsibilities" (ACA, 2014, p. 8).

Serving clients through a distance modality can affect us and fatigue us a lot. It can be tempting to roll from one online client meeting to the next with barely enough time for a "bio break." Instead, we need to take some real breaks and get ourselves in a centered and discerning space so that we can bring all our attention and energy to the screen, anticipate how clients experience us, and take care to develop their trust in our keen perceptiveness. We need to get even more prepared for each session, having a purpose and a plan before we start. And we need to develop ways to support ourselves after sessions; ironically, working through distance modalities can be even more intimate and intense than in-person work. Sometimes this involves just shaking off some heightened energy in a brisk walk around the block, but sometimes we need help in figuring out the perplexing things that happen. The practice of seeking help in supervision early in our career is worth maintaining later, through peer professional support.

Ethical Decision-Making

Because making ethical decisions is so important, and yet sometimes so tricky, therapists have thoughtfully created roadmaps for working through the tricky (and sometimes alarming) issues we face in a profession where so much is at stake, both for us and for our clients. For this reason, several models or plans for working through issues have been developed by moral philosophers and thoughtful practitioners. One of the most practical and logical ones available was developed by Holly Forester-Miller and Thomas Davis (2016) and is available in full on the ACA's website.

In brief, here are the steps these authors suggest for working through an ethical issue. These can easily be applied to specific situations in telemental health:

1. Identify the problem.
2. Apply the ACA code of ethics (or the code of ethics most relevant to your practice).
3. Determine the nature and dimensions of the dilemma.
4. Generate potential courses of action.

5. Consider the potential consequences of all options and determine a course of action.
6. Evaluate the selected course of action. Here are three simple tests to help you in your evaluation:

    a. Justice: Would you treat others the same in this situation?
    b. Publicity: Would you want your actions/decision reported in the press?
    c. Universality: Would you recommend the same course of action to another counselor in the same situation?

7. Implement the course of action.

For an opportunity to practice your ethical decision-making skills, please see the hypothetical dilemmas involving the practice of telemental health following the summary.

VOICES FROM THE FIELD

How do ethical decision-making models help you as a LPC providing telemental health services?

"Use and documentation of an ethical decision-making model is a key element of ensuring that all relevant ethical, legal, professional, and clinical issues are being accounted for and all stakeholders are being considered with potential courses of action and outcomes. Telemental health is a relatively new part of our field, thus counselors are facing new and complex ethical dilemmas in delivering safe, effective, responsible services. Many of the ways counselors would have engaged ethically with clients in person do not directly translate to virtual settings, and it is important that the counselor be prepared to navigate inevitable ethical dilemmas. There are many ethical decision-making models available throughout the professional literature. Use and documentation of one of these models will ensure that the counselor is considering all applicable codes of ethics, laws, stakeholder consequences, and potentials for harm. It is also important to remember that all applicable codes of ethics must be considered, not only those specifying telemental health."

–Marisa Whitsett, M.A., LPC-MHSP, NCC, Memphis, TN

Chapter Summary

In concluding this chapter, we hope you have an increased appreciation for how ethical codes reflect the shared values of a profession and the role they play in guiding the behavior of its members. As you prepare to live out an ethical commitment and align your practice to the various code sections, remember that at a fundamental level their purpose is all the same. Our ethical codes bind us in what Albert Schweitzer described as a sense of solidarity with other human beings. They represent our commitment to promoting the health and safety of our clients and communities.

If you haven't already set up your virtual telemental health toolbox, consider taking that step now. Make bookmarking the code(s) of ethics for your profession(s) your first addition. Then identify the state or states in which you would like to practice and use the sites highlighted throughout the chapter to determine if reciprocity has been established for your field between the states, and if not, decide whether obtaining a second license or volunteering may be options. Next, research the licensing and telemental health regulations and other laws governing the privacy of PHI, limitations of confidentiality, and the processes and resources you will need to help your clients through mental health emergencies or situations when a client may be a risk to themselves or someone else. Remember, knowing we have a responsibility to protect our clients and the public, and knowing how to do that on short notice, requires different types of preparation! We recommend adding relevant websites and trackers to your virtual telemental health toolbox as you conduct your research.

In the spirit of a profession that rests on supervised practice, do challenge yourself to complete the activities throughout the chapter for practice resolving ethical dilemmas. You may even come up with some of your own, based on experiences shared in class, or as you imagine the client populations for which you may provide care at a distance. Take advantage of the experiences and wisdom of your colleagues in training, professors, and supervisors as you study, train, and move into independent practice. Consultation and collaboration are time-tested strategies when navigating ethical dilemmas. Plan to take good care of yourself; we must be well in order to help others effectively and ethically.

APPLICATION EXERCISE

Now that you have completed reading this chapter, we imagine you are wondering how you will ever remember all that you need to anticipate and prevent potential ethical and legal issues, both for your clients and yourself! We encourage you to remember that, as in all professional matters, the intricacies of staying out of ethical and legal trouble involves both *prevention* and *cure*. In other words, first consider *what can be done ahead of time to anticipate potential problems*, and if something goes awry, *what needs to be done now to mitigate problems or get things back on track*.

To give you some practice, work with other students to identify key ethical considerations in the hypothetical cases involving telemental health presented next. While identifying ethical violations or questionable practices, also identify practices that could have *prevented* issues from arising. Use Forester-Miller and Davis's steps in the "Ethical Decision-Making Model at a Glance" to identify the problem, apply the code of ethics, determine the nature and dimensions of the dilemma, generate potential courses of action, evaluate them, and choose one. In other words, decide what, specifically, needs to be done next. Compare notes with others and, if needed, revise your plan. Additionally, imagine you could help the counselor "roll back time" and put specific practices in place that would have prevented the problem from occurring. What would you include?

Kara and Luis: Telemental Health With a Teen

Luis has a private practice in which he works with children and adolescents. Luis did a lot of research and found a platform from which he provides counseling in live video calls through a secure, HIPAA-compliant telehealth application that has bank-level encryption for his practice management software. He entered a business associate agreement with the company.

Luis is on a list maintained by the local school district for private counseling referrals, a practice that recently became more common as the need for mental health care surpassed school resources. One referral he received was for Kara, a 14-year-old-client who was reported as having problems with school attendance due to anxiety. Luis obtained consent for treatment from Kara's parents and assent for treatment from Kara.

As part of the consent process, Luis emphasized and secured agreement from Kara's parents to have her counseling take place online, in a private place in their home. However, they only have one computer, which is used for work by Kara's mother; it is located in a family room that has no door. As there seemed to be no interruptions during the initial sessions with Kara, Luis assumed that confidentiality was assured. However, during the fourth session, Kara appears tense and gives only vague responses to Luis's questions. Luis notices that Kara's forehead looks bruised, but he is not sure. Kara holds up a note for him to read that says, "I can't talk. Can I text you? What's your phone number?" and then points to somewhere off screen while raising her eyebrows. Luis is perplexed; he is concerned about Kara. Suddenly, a younger child pops on the screen and yells, "Don't tell him! Don't tell him!" Kara appears to panic. The session ends as Luis's screen goes blank.

June and Cam: Online Possibilities

June runs an online support group for adults with loved ones who have chronic health conditions. For ease of the participants' use, June uses a popular meeting platform with which the group members have familiarity. Before initiating the group, she required a private meeting with each participant to ensure their appropriateness. During one of these meetings, she discovered that she had known one of the prospective participants, Cam, while they were in high school. But this was some time ago, and their relationship at the time had been casual, so June saw no problem including Cam in the group.

The group has an ongoing "rolling" admission policy, and while other group members have come and gone, Cam has stayed on. While June noticed this, she was not concerned; Cam was a good group member, never missing a session and always telling poignant stories about what was going on at home. June appreciated that Cam made the group sessions livelier for all.

One evening during the group, Cam wrote to June privately in the chat, requesting that they both stay on after the session closed. Puzzled but not concerned, June agreed to do so. When June and Cam were alone in the video room, Cam confessed to having strong—and longstanding—feelings for June. Cam even admitted to making "screen grabs" during their meetings and creating photos of June "to help [him] get through the day—because [he] experience[s her] as so calming and supportive." Cam then politely asked if it would be possible to shift from group therapy to private therapy so they could "go deeper."

Now it is your turn. Using Forester-Miller and Davis's (2016) model for ethical decision-making, review the dilemmas and work through the steps. First, identify the problem, then apply the code of ethics most relevant to your profession. State what you see as the nature and dimensions of the dilemma. Then generate potential courses of action, considering the possible consequences of each option. Finally, select your recommendations for actions to take.

Next, roll back the clock, prior to the day the counselor and the client had their first contact. Utilizing the resources provided throughout the chapter, consider these questions: What should have been in place that wasn't? What professional practices and ethical guidelines were missed? What resources might have helped the counselor practice more professionally?

SPOTLIGHT ON TELEMENTAL HEALTH AND ETHICS IN THE SCHOOL SETTING

Carmen Connelly Pangelinan, PhD
Professional School Counselor, Fairfax, VA

Going Virtual in a School Setting

As a professional school counselor in a K–6 school, I had to adapt my school-based counseling practices quickly when the COVID-19 pandemic forced schools to go virtual. The urgency of establishing effective strategies to support students via telehealth services was apparent, yet the overarching question of "how" to fundamentally prepare for and execute ethical and legal telehealth practice with students had to be answered. Spring of 2020 was a time of extraordinary deliberation for my colleagues and me.

While adhering to the same ethical standards as I would when working face-to-face, I had to establish new processes as I initiated my online service and established a virtual school-based telehealth program. Practical strategies included collaborating with teachers, students, and parents to identify student needs and to privately access students for services. Navigating through this transition was complex! My approach to ethical telehealth practice was pinned to the *2016 American School Counselor Association (ASCA) Ethical Standards for School Counselors* and the *2014 American Counseling Association (ACA) Code of Ethics*. I made a concerted effort to synthesize both sets of standards with particular emphasis on Section A.15 of the ASCA Ethical Standards (2016) and Section H of the ACA Code of Ethics (2014) to guide my work while protecting students' confidentiality and rights. Additionally, a supplemental piece of ethical guidance I applied is outlined in the *ASCA Professional Standards and Competencies* (2019); how was I to serve my school community within this new environment?

Developing and preserving the integrity of the counseling relationship was fundamentally critical, especially within the virtual space. I adapted the informed consent process for virtual practice and protected the confidentiality of my students who were now at home with their families. Fortunately, I was not alone in adapting my practice. Through collaboration with county representatives, I acquired an electronic version of parent consent. Vital to my services, the parent consent included information on the benefits and limitations of short-term distance counseling, one of the services I provide as a professional school counselor. Acknowledging the limitations to confidentiality within the virtual platform and taking the necessary precautions to protect student privacy was key. Just as I established a private space, students (and parents) were asked to do the same.

Another caveat of ethical consideration is the process of identifying and responding to immediate student needs. In collaboration with our administration, tech team, and school clinicians, I disseminated county-provided protocols for student-sensitive information to all staff and monitored all referred cases. Obtaining access to contact information for students, parents, clinical team members, administration, and community resources were imperative to my responsive services and our crisis response team.

References

American Association of Marriage and Family Therapists. (n.d.). *Coronavirus and state/provincial telehealth guidelines*. https://www.aamft.org/Events/State_Guide_for_Telehealth.aspx

American Counseling Association. (n.d.). *Students and telebehavioral health*. https://www.counseling.org/membership/aca-and-you/students

American Counseling Association. (n.d.). *Telebehavioral health information and counselors in health care*. https://www.counseling.org/knowledge-center/mental-health-resources/trauma-disaster/telehealth-information-and-counselors-in-health-care

American Counseling Association. (2014). *Code of ethics*. https://www.counseling.org/resources/aca-code-of-ethics.pdf

American Counseling Association. (2022). *State licensure boards that have adopted the ACA code of ethics*. https://www.counseling.org/docs/default-source/licensure/state-licensure-boards-that-have-adopted-the-aca-code-of-ethics-(pdf).pdf?sfvrsn=9331cb46_2

American Psychological Association. (2015). *What you need to know before choosing online therapy.* https://www.apa.org/topics/telehealth/online-therapy

Association for Counselor Education and Supervision. (2011). *Best practices in clinical supervision.* https://acesonline.net/wp-content/uploads/2018/11/ACES-Best-Practices-in-Clinical-Supervision-2011.pdf

Barnett, J. E., & Kolmes, K. (2016). The practice of tele-mental health: Ethical, legal, and clinical issues for practitioners. *Practice Innovations, 1*(1), 53–66. https://doi.org/10.1037/pri0000014

Bodulovic, G., de Morpurgo, M., & Saunders, E. J. (2020, November 19). *Telehealth around the world: A global guide.* DLA Piper. https://www.dlapiper.com/en/italy/insights/publications/2020/11/telehealth-around-the-world-global-guide/

Bologna, C. (2020, September 23). Is it OK to record your therapy sessions? *HuffPost.* https://www.huffpost.com/entry/record-therapy-sessions-ok_l_5f6a13c5c5b6968b276fb61f

Center for Credentialing & Education. (n.d.). *BC-TMH: Board-certified-telemental health provider.* https://www.cce-global.org/credentialing/bctmh

Center for Credentialing & Education. (2008). *The approved clinical supervisor (ACS) code of ethics.* https://www.ncblpc.org/Assets/LawsAndCodes/ACS_Code_of_Ethics(forSupervisors).pdf

Coffman, C., & Barnett, J. E. (2021). *Informed consent with children and adolescents.* Society for the Advancement of Psychotherapy. https://societyforpsychotherapy.org/informed-consent-with-children-and-adolescents/

Drum, K. B., & Littleton, H. L. (2014). Therapeutic boundaries in telepsychology: Unique issues and best practice recommendations. *Professional Psychology: Research and Practice, 45*(5), 309–315. https://doi.org/10.1037/a0036127

Forester-Miller, H., & Davis, T. E. (2016). *Practitioner's guide to ethical decision making* (rev. ed.). https://www.counseling.org/docs/default-source/ethics/practioner-39-s-guide-to-ethical-decision-making.pdf

Healthcare Providers Service Organization. (n.d.). *Counseling board complaint case study: Unprofessional conduct while providing services through a mental health therapy app.* https://www.hpso.com/Resources/Legal-and-Ethical-Issues/Counselor-Case-Study-Mental-Health-Therapy-App

Johnson, K. F., & Rehfuss, M. (2021). Telehealth interprofessional education: Benefits, desires, and concerns of counselor trainees. *Journal of Creativity in Mental Health, 16*(1), 15–30. https://doi.org/10.1080/15401383.2020.1751766

Lerman, A., & Ozinal, F. R. (2021, November 18). *Just released: Telemental health laws – download our complimentary survey/app and learn more.* https://www.healthlawadvisor.com/2021/11/18/just-released-telemental-health-laws-download-our-complimentary-survey-app-and-learn-more/

Lively, T. K. (2022, April 28). *US state privacy legislation tracker.* International Association of Privacy Professional. https://iapp.org/resources/article/us-state-privacy-legislation-tracker/

Lloyd-Hazlett, J., & Foster, V. A. (2017). Student counselors' moral, intellectual, and professional ethical identity development. *Counseling and Values, 62*(1), 90–105. https://doi.org/10.1002/cvj.12051

Luxton, D. D., Nelson, E. L., & Maheu, M. M. (2016). A practitioner's guide to telemental health: How to conduct legal, ethical, and evidence-based telepractice. American Psychological Association. https://doi.org/10.1037/14938-000

Machuca, R., & Kurns, A. (2021). The virtual bug: Online live supervision of telemental health counseling. *Journal of Technology in Counselor Education and Supervision, 1*(1), 3–15.

Martin, L. (2019). Before you press record. California Association of Marriage and Family Therapists. https://www.camft.org/Resources/Legal-Articles/Chronological-Article-List/before-you-press-record

McKnight-Lizotte, M. (2020). A practitioner's guide to telemental health: How to conduct legal, ethical, and evidence-based telepractice. *Best Practices in Mental Health, 16*(2), 71–73.

Meyers, L. (2014, May 22). A living document of ethical guidance. *Counseling Today.* https://ct.counseling.org/2014/05/a-living-document-of-ethical-guidance/

Meyers, L. (2018, April 30). #disconnected: Why counselors can no longer ignore social media. *Counseling Today.* https://ct.counseling.org/2018/04/disconnected-why-counselors-can-no-longer-ignore-social-media/

National Alliance for Caregiving and American Association of Retired Persons. (2020). *Caregiving in the U.S. 2020.* https://www.caregiving.org/caregiving-in-the-us-2020/

National Center for Interstate Counseling Compacts. (2022). *Counseling Compact.* https://counselingcompact.org/

National Center on Disability and Access to Education. (2022). *NCDAE tips and tools: Principles of accessible design.* https://ncdae.org/resources/factsheets/principles.php

Office for Civil Rights. (2021). *HIPAA for professionals.* U.S. Department of Health and Human Services. https://www.hhs.gov/hipaa/for-professionals/index.html

Office of the National Coordinator for Health Information Technology. (n.d.). *Guide to privacy and security of health information* https://www.healthit.gov/sites/default/files/pdf/privacy/onc_privacy_and_security_chapter4_v1_022112.pdf

Phillips, L. (2022, March 25). The rise of counselors on social media. *Counseling Today.* https://ct.counseling.org/2022/03/the-rise-of-counselors-on-social-media/?utm_source=listeningpost&utm_medium=email&utm_campaign=ctonline&utm_term=article&utm_content=counselorsonsocial

Psychology.org Staff. (2022, January 19). *Virtual therapy vs. in-person therapy.* Psychology.org. https://www.psychology.org/resources/virtual-therapy-vs-in-person/

Ratts, M., Singh, A., Nassar-McMillan, S., Butler, K., & McCullough, J. R. (2016). *Multicultural and social justice counseling competencies.* https://doi.org/10.13140/RG.2.1.1989.8002

Reinhardt, R. (2019, January 16). Technology tutor: Taking a closer look at telehealth. *Counseling Today.* https://ct.counseling.org/2019/01/technology-tutor-taking-a-closer-look-at-telehealth/

Schaffer, C. T., Nakrani, P., Pirraglia, P. A. (2020). Telemental health care: A review of efficacy and interventions. *Telehealth and Medicine Today, 5*(4). https://doi.org/10.30953/tmt.v5.218

Stoll, J., Muller, J. A., & Trachsel, M. (2020). Ethical issues in online psychotherapy: A narrative review. *Frontiers in Psychiatry, 10,* 1–16. https://doi.org/10.3389/fpsyt.2019.00993

Telebehavioral Health Institute, Inc. (2017). *The telebehavioral health informed consent library.* https://www.naadac.org/assets/2416/marlene_maheu_ac17h02.pdf

Telehealth Certification Institute. (2022). *States' telemental health laws, rules, and regulations.* https://www.telementalhealthtraining.com/states-rules-and-regulations

U.S. Department of Health and Human Services. (n.d.). *The HIPAA privacy rule.* https://www.hhs.gov/hipaa/for-professionals/privacy/index.html

U.S. Department of Health and Human Services. (2021). *Legal considerations.* https://telehealth.hhs.gov/providers/legal-considerations/

World Wide Web Consortium. (2022). *Web accessibility initiative.* https://www.w3.org/WAI/

Wrape, E. R., & McGinn, M. M. (2019). Clinical and ethical considerations for delivering couple and family therapy via telehealth. *Journal of Marital & Family Therapy, 45*(2), 296–308. https://doi.org/10.1111/jmft.12319

Yalom, I. D., & Yalom, M. (2021). *A matter of life and death.* Stanford University Press.

CHAPTER 3

Technical and Practical Considerations for Telemental Health

Nicole M. Arcuri Sanders

Failing to prepare is preparing to fail.

–Benjamin Franklin

Learning Objectives

After reading this chapter, you should be able to do the following:

- Identify ethical and legal responsibilities to technical and practical considerations related to telemental health services
- Apply ethical codes and state statutes when creating your telemental health counseling space
- Analyze personal-professional presentation
- Examine personal-professional communication
- Design a professional counseling space for telemental health services

Introduction

Telemental health practices have been available for years; however, the necessity for application was not apparent until more recently with the COVID-19 pandemic. As early as the 1920s, medical centers conducted medical consultations for remote islands and those on ships in Europe (Ryu, 2010). Later, the United States introduced organized telemedicine programs in the 1950s. Years later, in 2016, research found that telehealth was on the rise due to ease of access, providing clients with convenience, the ability to address more diagnoses, and the migration of telehealth to mobile devices; however, widespread use by many was restricted due to limited reimbursement by third-party payers (e.g., insurance companies) (Ray & Topol, 2016). Additional factors impacting the limited use of telehealth services included concerns for quality care, social stigma, and legal and ethical uncertainties. However, when countries shut down due to the COVID-19 global pandemic, state licensure and practice laws had to quickly address the needs of their clients by implementing telehealth services to support continuity of care and ensure clients were not abandoned or neglected (American Counseling Association [ACA], 2014, A.12.).

During this time, many counselors were unfamiliar and untrained to address the increasing mental health needs of the population via a telehealth platform. The Centers for Disease Control and Prevention (CDC) reported increased symptoms of anxiety and depressive disorders during the pandemic, with anxiety disorder increasing approximately three times and the prevalence of depressive disorder approximately four times during April to June of 2020 compared to that same time period in 2019 (Czeisler et al., 2020). In this chapter, you will learn about technology implications to consider when you are getting started in telemental health and be provided with guidance to support you in your preparation for conducting counseling sessions from various distance modalities.

Technical Check-Up Before Practice

Whether you intend to provide telemental health services to your clients or are considering preparation in the event of an emergency situation (e.g., COVID-19), many ponder numerous questions concerning where to start. The first thing you want to do is check with your state licensure board to examine state laws relevant to telemental health services. Take it from someone who has their license in multiple states prior to COVID-19; these boards are imperative for you to stay up to date with! States vary

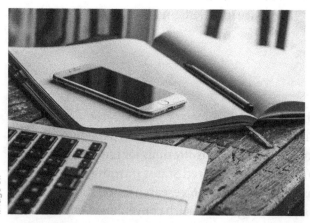

Image 3.1

on licensed practice laws; understanding what is allowed where and how is a necessity to ensure you maintain your credential. Additionally, as the needs of the world change, states sometimes have to provide emergency guidance based on federal government direction. If you ever have a question concerning a policy, it will be important to seek clarification directly from your state board. Once you feel confident in understanding what you are allowed to do and not do, you are ready to consider your technology needs.

Technology considerations can be overwhelming for many due to the constant and rapid advancements that take place. As time continues to evolve it is important to stay abreast of improvements in technology to offer your clients the best and most current services. For instance, think back to the 1950s when telehealth was being used and how much technological capabilities have changed since then! You want to also make sure you are aware of the clients you will be serving to ensure your technological modalities are accessible to them. Let's get started!

Privacy/Security

You might think that the removal of a client walking into an actual physical counseling office may provide the client with more protection when they can obtain counseling services from the confines of their own home; however, this is incorrect. This is equally true for the clinician. When the clinician brings their office to their home, additional safety measures need to be taken into consideration.

First, consider your setting. Your home is often your comfort zone where you can let loose and unwind. However, when bringing your profession into your home, it is imperative as a counselor to ensure you are able to establish and maintain professional boundaries with your clients (ACA, 2014, H.4.b.). With that being said, you want to be mindful of what you showcase to your client; remember that the session is intended to explore the needs of the client. Of course, it can be nice to have a client get a sense of who you authentically and genuinely are, but this can be done by ensuring that your personal belongings are not in camera view (e.g., laundry, including undergarments). I personally have always been lucky enough to have at least a small nook for privacy. However, I've had colleagues, supervisees, as well as clients share with me events that they wish they could have avoided over the years. For instance, I had a colleague who at one time did not know their spouse had to pick up their sick child from daycare. All was fine until the client got a glimpse of the spouse changing their child's diaper in the background. Despite the closed office they had, which provided them volume privacy, they quickly learned that the glass door did not offer visual privacy. I share this as a learning opportunity for us all, as mistakes are rich lessons for growth!

Some of you may be thinking, "How will I do this if I live in what already feels like a cramped home?" Why not consider dedicating a small corner specifically devoted to your work using a temporary wall partition? You can also take additional steps to ensure privacy of conversations with additional items such as earphones/pods as well as ensure that others are not in earshot of the office (e.g., children, spouse/partner, family member, roommate).

Not only should you be concerned with the privacy you offer within a telemental health session due to ethical and legal implications connected to confidentiality, but also for considerations of safety. Screening clients for suitability to online counseling and safety concerns is a key step and will be discussed further in Chapter 5. Remember that despite all the steps one may take to screen clients, we are all susceptible to work with violent clients in our careers. Therefore, counselors need to monitor self-disclosure. Ultimately, we are inviting clients into our virtual home office, and it is imperative for counselors to maintain professional boundaries that do not put themselves or others who live with them in danger. I often share with my supervisees the following: Most people do not attend counseling because they cannot wait to tell you just how wonderful things are going in their life. They are there because they are experiencing some discomfort in life that is creating a disequilibrium for them. This discomfort can sometimes support unpredictable and irrational behaviors as they try to gain a sense of stability. Therefore, your safety as a counselor must always be considered. When in your home, the safety of those in your personal life, such as your loved ones, also needs to be considered.

When considering others in your home, you must be mindful of having pictures of your children, family, and friends in the background. It is important to check with the individuals in the photo to make sure they are comfortable with this being shared with your clients. For instance, if you live with a partner and your child, is your partner be okay with your clients seeing a picture of you and them on a family vacation? Is your child comfortable with this? Are you comfortable with this? The same may be true for your client. Clients may or may not be comfortable with sharing certain aspects of their life, and furthermore, those who reside with them may not be comfortable with it. I've had many supervisees inquire about whether this type of disclosure is beneficial. There is a great deal of research to support therapeutic rapport being a paramount component to client success. A counselor being genuine and authentic can alone be therapeutic for clients (Rogers, 1957); however, this does not mean that a counselor and/or their loved one's safety should ever be jeopardized.

Also, students have inquired whether a client hiding aspects of their life may be an indication of a client who is not ready to change. This may be true for some. However, remember that we are asking clients to meet with us, a stranger, and become vulnerable. Think about when you first meet a stranger—do you feel comfortable sharing everything about you? The same is true for our clients. When stepping into our counseling office, they have the opportunity to come to a space that is safe and nonjudgmental, offering them an opportunity to share aspects of their lives that they may have never shared with anyone else. For some clients, their home may be a place that is adding to their experience of disequilibrium in their life. Clients have the right to keep some aspects personal and to protect the confidentiality and privacy of others in their space as well. Trust takes time, and with time clients tend to open up more, which may mean that they may invite more of their personal space into their sessions when they are ready.

As alluded to earlier, this space must also be free from others to promote confidentiality. If I was conducting a session and my husband walked by in the background, whether I had a headset on or not, this could make my client feel vulnerable that perhaps another person (who is not their counselor) saw them on the screen or may have overheard them at some point. Remember, counselors

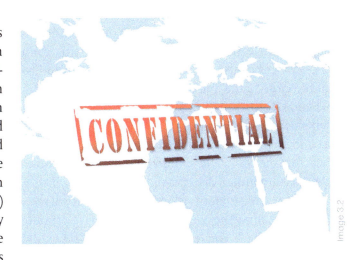

cannot ethically verify to others if any of their clients is actually their client without the written permission of their client/client's guardian or the client disclosing willingly, without coercion, to another. Counselors are ethically responsible to respect the confidentiality of clients (ACA, 2014, B.1.a) and provide the client with a confidential counseling setting (B.3.c). Therefore, when conducting telemental health services from your home, the counselor will want to take precautions to provide their clients with a confidential space that is intended to be free of interruptions during the duration of the session. Counselors are encouraged to explore this notion of a safe space with clients as well to support honest, open, and active participation by the clients. If the client has someone else present in their home who may be able to overhear the session, the client may not be open and honest. Therefore, ensuring a client is alone, free from distractions, and expresses who is in the room should be confirmed between counselor and client. Camera placement is also important for all parties involved in the session.

What should be in your camera's lens? As the counselor, you want to check with your state board concerning licensure and degree display requirements. Most states require your credential to be visible to your clients at all times of services. If this is the case in your state, you want to ensure your credential can be seen. Additionally, consider your style based on your professional disclosure statement that provides an open, nonjudgmental, and inviting space to clients in general (since everyone is unique and will vary in preferences).

Personally, I have my credentials in the background, a large picture of a sun setting over a bay, and the space to move my chair toward and away from the screen so that I can mirror my clients when needed or demonstrate certain interventions (e.g., dance movement strategies, deep breathing, empty chair, muscle relaxation). By allowing your client to see more than just your face, you can introduce nonverbal mirroring and interventions. Additionally, by showing more of yourself, your clients may be more inclined to do the same so that you as the counselor can be more in-tune to how they are presenting as a whole (e.g., hygiene, nonverbals). For some, this may be limiting due to technology availability.

However, the increasing production of various Bluetooth earphones with microphone capabilities (e.g., AirPods) are supporting this ability more readily. Such technology accessories can also support the concern with audio capabilities with telehealth. If you sit too close to the mic on your computer/tablet/phone, the voice may appear too loud, whereas if you are far away it may be difficult to hear you. This is an attribute a counselor will need to practice prior to a session to ensure they are familiar with their space as well as camera lens and microphone capabilities. If a client indicates they are having difficulty hearing, the counselor should be familiar with how to quickly troubleshoot to ensure the least amount of disruption to counseling services (ACA, 2014, C.2.).

The next consideration concerns the clarity of the view. Ask yourself, "Does the space I am using allow the client to see me clearly without sun glare or shadows due to being in a dark space?" You really do not want to be a silhouette for your client! You want to ensure your space has adequate lighting that allows you to remain visible for the entirety of the session. For instance, where my office is located, depending on the season, there is about a 35-minute period where I need to ensure my blinds are shut and the lamps are on to avoid changing light variations with the sun setting. However, this choice may bring additional considerations related to internet capabilities. Some rooms may have better capabilities than others. You want to ensure you can support uninterrupted sessions from your space. This may take some trial-and-error experiences on your behalf, but you want to do this prior to your first client session. I am not saying that technological difficulties may not still be experienced along the way. We cannot control everything (e.g., weather, power/internet outage), but we need to plan to minimize interruptions to our clients and to have back-up plans in the event an interruption does occur. The point of focusing on clarity of view is to stress the importance of you appearing confident and competent in using the modality in your space. If in numerous sessions you spend most of your time troubleshooting, this can distract from the counseling process.

Clients should feel supported by their counselor from the start with the establishment of a space ready to effectively offer counseling services; counselors need to ethically demonstrate knowledge and competency in their delivery efforts (ACA, 2014, H.1.a). There may be some events that a counselor cannot prevent (e.g., natural disasters, large outages), but the counselor should ethically account for this possibility and ensure their clients are aware of back-up plans when there are technology failures (H.2.a). This should be addressed within the informed consent prior to commencing services with clients.

Professional Presentation

> If you don't know what you want to achieve in your presentation your audience never will."
>
> *–Harvey Diamond*

I ask you to consider this quote and then ask yourself these questions:

- How do you want to be received by your client?
- What type of feeling do you hope your client gets when first entering a session with you?
- What are you wearing? What are you not wearing?
- What is in your background? What is not in your background?
- How much of "you" does your client see in the camera view?

Knowing the impression you want your client to have of you to sets the tone of your counseling therapeutic relationship and is imperative prior to commencing services. This should be considered an important part of your professional identity and theoretical orientation. Now that you are ready to begin working with clients, how do you want to be received? As noted earlier, you want your clients to see you as competent in your professional role as a counselor and as capable to conduct services using distance platforms. Just as if you were working with clients in a brick-and-mortar face-to-face setting, the digital space you invite them into matters. Is the room cluttered with client files everywhere or are confidential materials out of view? Can the client focus on you and your conversation or are there distracting contents in the room? Does the space offer them a place to think and speak at the volume they choose or are they talking over loud noises? Are others able to overhear your session or do clients see you as providing them with a confidential space? These are some of the many details that counselors can take for granted when they get ready for work and turn on the computer.

VOICES FROM THE FIELD

What was your experience like transitioning to a telemental health practice?

"I got certified in 2015 when I was working with patients. I knew the field was headed this way. I wasn't expecting a pandemic but I knew that telehealth was going to be the new normal."
    –Fredrick Dombrowski, PhD, LMHC, CASAC, LPC, LADC, NCC, CCMHC, MAC, ACS, BC-TMH, HS-BCP, ICADC, DCMHS, Milford, CT

"I am in a rural area where public transportation is not readily available and in winter travel is difficult. COVID-19 increased the requests for online therapy, so it was important for me to increase access. The client is asked to be in a secluded room and I sit in my office with the doors closed and white noise playing in the waiting room while doing telemental health. I have used blue jeans with students connected to school-based internet, VSEE and purchased Zoom (confidential) with clients."

    –Cheryl Welch, PhD, LPC, RN, Florence, WI

"I wanted to have a way to continue to practice. I am a Counselor Educator and want to continue to experience providing counseling in order to relate to my students. I stopped counseling for a couple of years and realized with teaching my students that I missed the rewarding aspect of counseling not to mention to relate more to my student's experiences. I think that clients are going to demand more telemental health in the future and the licensure governing bodies need to figure out a way to make it so licenses have more portability."

–Alice Crawford, LCPC, Carpentersville, IL

"I transitioned to full telehealth services March 13, 2020 due to COVID lockdown. I participated in a PESI telehealth training and researched ethical obligations for telehealth as well as HIPAA compliant platforms, informed consents for the telehealth platform, changed my Psychology Today profile to state offering of telehealth services. At first, I started with my laptop at my kitchen table, which did not work for long. I brought a table from my therapy office home to set up a desk in my dining room and purchased a desktop computer as I started having issues with weary eyes because of the blue light. I have thoroughly enjoyed telehealth."

–Kelly James, PhD, LPC, NCC, Tulsa, OK

Counseling Space

Since you will be the person in charge of designing the counseling space (e.g., home-based telehealth counselor), these questions must be examined. So once again I ask you, how do you want your clients to see you? I encourage you to take a moment and process the questions in the previous section. Consider what you want your counseling space to look like in your home. Where will it be? Do you need to change anything to that area now? Remember it does not need to be a whole room, but a place during specific times of your sessions where this space will not be interrupted. How will you do that? Maybe you feel the need to get up and actually tour your space and try to create this space now. Maybe you are deciding to Google *home office looks*. Whatever you are doing to start the process of assessing the space you want to invite your clients into, remember your ethical and legal requirements as a professional counselor (e.g., boundaries, confidentiality, credentialing display, security, technology accessibility). In Table 3.1, you will find ACA (2014) codes of ethics that should be considered when designing your counseling space. The ACA code of ethics was examined in more detail in Chapter 2. The purpose of this table is to propose questions to consider in helping you create an ethical telemental health space for your clients. Consider the questions and record your responses on your own for reflection.

TABLE 3.1 Counseling Space Ethical and Legal Analysis Chart

ACA (2014) Code	Question(s)
BOUNDARIES	
H.4.b. Professional Boundaries in Distance Counseling Counselors understand the necessity of maintaining a professional relationship with their clients. Counselors discuss and establish professional boundaries with clients regarding the appropriate use and/or application of technology and the limitations of its use within the counseling relationship (e.g., lack of confidentiality, times when not appropriate to use).	▪ Do the clients see pictures of you and your family/friends in other roles? ▪ Do you have personal calendars viewable? ▪ Are personal/social invitations viewable? ▪ Does the space offer a distraction-free setting that supports the well-being of the client first and foremost (A.1.a)? Are you impaired due to distractions (e.g., room-mate, spouse, child, cleaning service, repair person, etc.; C.2.g)
RECORDS AND CONFIDENTIALITY	
A.1.b. Records and Documentation Counselors create, safeguard, and maintain documentation necessary for rendering professional services. Regardless of the medium, counselors include sufficient and timely documentation to facilitate the delivery and continuity of services. Counselors take reasonable steps to ensure that documentation accurately reflects client progress and services provided. If amendments are made to records and documentation, counselors take steps to properly note the amendments according to agency or institutional policies. **B.1.c. Respect for Confidentiality** Counselors protect the confidential information of prospective and current clients. Counselors disclose information only with appropriate consent or with sound legal or ethical justification. **B.3.c. Confidential Settings** Counselors discuss confidential information only in settings in which they can reasonably ensure client privacy. **B.6.b. Confidentiality of Records and Documentation** Counselors ensure that records and documentation kept in any medium are secure and that only authorized persons have access to them.	▪ Where are client case notes and files? Are they viewable to your clients? ▪ Can you clients view your case notes, files, billing, or any other documentation? ▪ Can anyone else in the home/setting access the records and documentation? If so, do they have permission to do so? ▪ Where are current, past, and future client documentation stored? Who has access? ▪ How do you dispose of documentation? Is it secure? ▪ What happens to your documentation in the event you are unable to return to work? Do you have a professional will? Who has access to your records if you die or become incapacitated (spouse, children)? ▪ Is the platform only accessible to your client? Can other clients access it? What security measures have you taken to ensure only your client has access to their session?

(Continued)

ACA (2014) Code	Question(s)
RECORDS AND CONFIDENTIALITY	
B.6.h. Storage and Disposal After Termination Counselors store records following termination of services to ensure reasonable future access, maintain records in accordance with federal and state laws and statutes such as licensure laws and policies governing records, and dispose of client records and other sensitive materials in a manner that protects client confidentiality. Counselors apply careful discretion and deliberation before destroying records that may be needed by a court of law, such as notes on child abuse, suicide, sexual harassment, or violence. **B.6.i. Reasonable Precautions** Counselors take reasonable precautions to protect client confidentiality in the event of the counselor's termination of practice, incapacity, or death and appoint a records custodian when identified as appropriate.	
STATE GUIDANCE	
H.1.b. Laws and Statutes Counselors who engage in the use of distance counseling, technology, and social media within their counseling practice understand that they may be subject to laws and regulations of both the counselor's practicing location and the client's place of residence. Counselors ensure that their clients are aware of pertinent legal rights and limitations governing the practice of counseling across state lines or international boundaries.	• Do you have to display your counseling credential(s)? • Can your office travel (e.g., tiny home on wheels)? If so, are there any boundaries that need to be considered?
VALUES	
A.4.b. Personal Values Counselors are aware of—and avoid imposing—their own values, attitudes, beliefs, and behaviors. Counselors respect the diversity of clients, trainees, and research participants and seek training in areas in which they are at risk of imposing their values onto clients, especially when the counselor's values are inconsistent with the client's goals or are discriminatory in nature.	• Does your space indicate your values? Can it be offensive to others? Does anything in this space suggest you are possibly imposing a value onto your clients?

ACA (2014) Code	Question(s)
VALUES	
B.1.a. Multicultural/Diversity Considerations Counselors maintain awareness and sensitivity regarding cultural meanings of confidentiality and privacy. Counselors respect differing views toward disclosure of information. Counselors hold ongoing discussions with clients as to how, when, and with whom information is to be shared.	• Is your space culturally considerate? Does your space intentionally create offense to others?

Counselor Professional Appearance

Now that you have considered your virtual counseling space, how will you be professionally viewed by your client while on screen? We discussed this a bit earlier in the chapter; however, professional presentation should be given specific consideration. At this point in the chapter, you may be feeling that the questions you need to ask of yourself to prepare for offering telemental health services to clients are endless; however, I encourage you to refrain from this thought and consider "What other questions should I be asking?" The reason for this is that we benefit most when we are intentionally postured for continued learning growth. Wouldn't you rather be prepared to address a concern than feel ill-equipped? If you don't have the answer, remember that is okay. We are a profession that supports one another in ongoing professional development, consultation, and supervision. In fact, even if you make a mistake along the way, but you take these ethical steps, you have shown intention to provide best practices for your client.

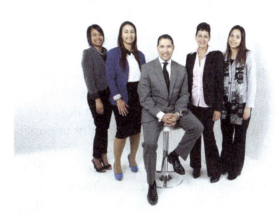

Image 3.3

Why is one's appearance important? Let's start by considering the mental status examination. There is a reason for a counselor to explore how a client presents (i.e., appearance). Basic grooming and hygiene can tell a lot about how a person is caring for themselves, which can provide insight concerning the severity of symptomology (e.g., depression, hopelessness). Appearance changes can also highlight if improvements or regressions need to be considered. Consider if a client sees you come to session with your hair unkept, dirt on your face, and appearing as if you have not slept in days. What type of comfort do you believe they will have in your services? It is imperative that you as a counselor provide the client with an opportunity where they believe you can genuinely be in the moment and concerned with their well-being. Such an appearance can insinuate that you may need to work on yourself. For instance, if you are too tired, can you really focus on them during their session? If you appear alert and groomed, an idea that you are present and ready can be insinuated. With someone who has provided telemental health services while having an infant and toddler, I can understand that some days are harder than others to hide the sleepless night you just had. However, this is where you as a professional need to practice self-awareness and refrain from offering or providing professional services when impaired (ACA, 2014, C.2.g).

Something that I wish was shared with me during my graduate experience was the idea of matching my clients. We spend a great deal of time during graduate programs considering congruence of skills but not about our personal appearance. What I mean by this is if you are working with a homeless population and are dressed like you are attending a red-carpet event, can you be setting up an invisible boundary for such a drastic difference of economic means with the client? We discuss client–therapist match a great deal in case conceptualization, but this should also be considered with your appearance concerning dress. I am not saying that you need to mimic your clients exactly, but you should be cognizant of possible gaps you can be creating with your clients. For instance, when I work with clients who are in the business world, I try to present in business-professional attire as well. However, if I have a client who is a blue-collar worker, I attempt to come to the session more business casual. The difference from one session to the next may simply be putting on a suit jacket or tie. The clothing will also need to be appropriate for the type of interventions the counselor will be using. For instance, when incorporating dance movement, I need to be cognizant of how my clothing will shift with movement. Furthermore, if I am working with children, even virtually, sometimes I ask them to get comfortable and they sit on the floor. To help them feel okay with their decision, I too, sometimes sit on the floor in a more relaxed form. I need to be aware of what I am wearing so I can make these movements rather seamlessly and not distract from the session. So, consider the saying "dress for success" when you get ready for a telehealth session, but remember that dressing for success can look different for varying populations. This, again, is an aspect that highlights the idea that it is important to know who your clients are.

Counselor Professional Communication

Meeting your clients where they are also requires you to ensure your language matches their developmental as well as cognitive capabilities (ACA, 2014, A.2.c). However, I caution you to remember that your conversational manner should still support your role as a counselor (A.5 and A.6); you are not their friend venting about life. Therefore, you need to still be mindful of understanding how to professionally communicate in various formats while also considering their cognitive and developmental needs.

Furthermore, counselors should communicate in a culturally sensitive manner (A.2.c). This will again vary per the unique cognitive and developmental needs of clients as well as perception of their culture. For instance, I have provided counseling services to numerous clients within the military- and veteran-connected population. This culture uses a great deal of acronyms. This means that I not only need to be familiar with those acronyms but also know how to utilize them in my dialogue. I have had many clients over the years say something similar to me: "Next month we are expected to PCS, but we are still waiting to hear back from EFMP to see if my son will have the accommodations at the new station. This means we will have to do a DITY move." For those not familiar with the culture, this may make no sense, but in fact, it is a very concise statement that highlights the clarity of thought the client currently has. The client is sharing that they have received orders to move, known as PCS, which means a permanent change of station. They are currently unsure if the new location will be able to meet the needs of their son. Their son receives services from the Exceptional Family Member Program (EFMP). To qualify for this program, the person needs to have a physical, emotional, developmental, or intellectual disorder requiring specialized services. In the case that the station cannot meet the needs, the service member can file a waiver. However, the waiver can also be denied, which may result in the service member receiving orders separate from their family member(s), known as dependents. Due to this uncertainty, the family has chosen to move themselves to their next station because they may not have time to have the government move them. A DITY move is a personally procured move, also known as a do-it yourself move. Every culture and even subcultures within the culture have their own language and style of communication. This needs to be considered when working with all clients receiving telemental health services just as it would with brick-and-mortar face-to-face sessions. However, you may need to be especially mindful of this consideration if using text-based telemental health services.

Counselors providing telemental health services should be mindful of both synchronous (e.g., live) and asynchronous (e.g., time-delay) communications. When using video, both verbal and nonverbal communication need to be considered. Furthermore, the counselor needs to assess the client's intellectual, emotional, physical, linguistic, and functional capability of using the application and that the application is appropriate for the needs of the client (H.4.c). As discussed in Chapter 2, whether using video, audio phone, text messaging, or chat (synchronous, asynchronous) distance modalities, the counselor has the ethical responsibility to "use current encryption standards within their websites and/or technology-based communications that meet applicable legal requirements. Counselors take reasonable precautions to ensure the confidentiality of information transmitted through any electronic means" (ACA, 2014, H.2.d, p. 18). Counselors have to be especially mindful of clients' protected health information (PHI; e.g., birthday, phone number, diagnosis, address) during their communications as well since there are limits to confidentiality when using third-party systems. According to the Health Insurance Portability and Accountability Act (HIPAA), there are 18 personal identifiers. You want to limit the communication to what is therapeutically necessary. For instance, if using email to schedule/reschedule client sessions, you want to be mindful of client-identifying information shared in that email. Considering this, mental health professionals should use in-transit encryption (Elhai & Frueh, 2016). This means you get confirmation when you send an email to a client, when a client accesses, as well as when they read an email. However, a counselor should always remind their clients with the informed consent the limitations of confidentiality associated with technology (H.2.c). To minimize threats of breach of confidentiality (e.g., advertisements, hacks, apps with tracking access), it is suggested that counselors use end-to-end encryption of text messages by default. However, despite claims of HIPAA-compliant technologies (e.g., Apple's messages to other iOS users or smartphone apps such as Signal), counselors are still encouraged to de-identify information when transmitted using text-messaging capability (Lustgarten, 2020). The same is true for when using chat areas within a HIPAA-compliant videoconferencing platform (e.g., Zoom Business, Webex Business, Doxy.me). Please know these examples are shared in accordance with current standards; however, with the ever-evolving technological advances, it is important to stay current on federal and state requirements as well as changes to platforms.

Something to consider when using any platform is the security of the technology you are using (e.g., computer, tablet, smartphone). This highlights the need to protect data in transit as well as at rest. Your computer needs to be password protected. If saving data onto your hard drive, you need to ensure it is encrypted. Otherwise, you need to use an encrypted cloud-based service (e.g., SimplePractice). Smartphones and tablets also need to be encrypted per HIPAA regulations. Additional considerations are that you need to be on a password-protected router or use a virtual private network (VPN) when using other wireless routers (e.g., when traveling). As a side note, you want to remember to consider the state practicing laws of where you travel).

HIPAA compliance can appear overwhelming when considering the numerous steps the counselor needs to take to best protect clients. A great resource to help counselors build confidence with navigating what HIPAA guidelines really mean and how to implement them with confidence is called the HIPAA Guide (2021). Additionally, with the recent pandemic, many state licensing boards are also providing guidance concerning HIPAA compliance.

Remember that you are not alone in navigating telemental health services. As counselors, we are ethically responsible to seek consultation and supervision with areas in question, so don't be afraid to ask for guidance and/or to process your thoughts with your supervisors and colleagues. In fact, in the counseling field, this is invited, welcomed, and celebrated! Moreover, the field requires counselors to have ongoing training. There are numerous mental health training vendors who can aid you with additional support for building confidence with implementing ethical and legal telemental health services. In fact, you may want to check with your state board to see if they suggest any specific providers. Often these trainings are designed to address state requirements.

Chapter Summary

There is a great deal of thought that goes into the creation of a counseling space. As technology continues to evolve, counselors have the ethical responsibility to seek training to ensure they can provide clients with competent services that offer best practices while safeguarding both the counselor and the client. With that being said, counselors need to continuously self-monitor their effectiveness as well as evaluate the effectiveness of platforms. When and if an impairment is identified, the counselor has the ethical duty to address this. Years ago, I could have never imagined our field to be faced with a global pandemic, but now that it has, the event should prompt counselors to know where to turn to when exploring uncharted territories so that we can grow as professionals and provide our clients with best services despite the challenges. Remember that you do not need to memorize all the details outlined in this chapter, but it is important for a future professional counselor to have guidance with the technical and practical considerations of setting up a telemental health practice. When in doubt, seek supervision and/or consultation. We can only grow stronger as a profession through professional counselors' self-awareness, inquiry, evolution, professional development, and evaluation of effectiveness, as well as by addressing areas in need of enhancement. If in doubt, ask!

PERSONAL REFLECTION ACTIVITY

Your Virtual Counseling Space Design: In the box provided, visualize your future counseling space (you may want to make copies as your vision will likely transform over time).

Feel free to draw out, cut and paste a picture, and/or list important aspects concerning your home-based telehealth counseling space. Perhaps it is not in the residence you live now, but one where you are hopeful to practice one day!

References

American Counseling Association. (2014). *2014 ACA code of ethics.* Author.

Czeisler, M. É., Lane, R. I., Petrosky, E., Wiley, J. F., Christensen, A., Njai, R., Weaver, M. D., Robbins, R., Facer-Childs, E. R., Barger, L. K., Czeisler, C. A., Howard, M. E., & Rajaratnam, S. M. W. (2020). Mental health, substance use, and suicidal ideation during the COVID-19 pandemic—United States, June 24–30, 2020. *MMWR Morbidity and Mortality Weekly Report, 69*(32), 1049–1057. http://doi.org/10.15585/mmwr.mm6932a1

Elhai, J. D., & Frueh, B. C. (2016). Security of electronic mental health communication and record-keeping in the digital age. *Journal of Clinical Psychiatry, 77*(2), 262–268. http://doi.org/10.4088/jcp.14r09506

HIPAA Guide. (2021). *HIPAA compliance guide.* https://www.hipaaguide.net/hipaa-compliance-guide/

Lustgarten, S. D., Garrison, Y. L., Sinnard, M. T., & Flynn, A. W. (2020). Digital privacy in mental healthcare: Current issues and recommendations for technology use. *Current opinion in psychology, 36,* 25–31. https://doi.org/10.1016/j.copsyc.2020.03.012

Ray, D. E., & Topol, E. J. (2016). State of telehealth. *The New England Journal of Medicine, 375*(2), 154–161. http://doi.org/10.1056/NEJMra1601705

Rogers, C. R. (1957). The necessary and sufficient conditions of therapeutic personality change. *Journal of Consulting Psychology, 21*(2), 95–103. https://doi.org/10.1037/h0045357

Ryu, S. (2010). History of telemedicine: Evolution, context, and transformation. *Healthcare Informatics Research, 16*(1), 65–66. https://doi.org/10.4258/hir.2010.16.1.65

CHAPTER 4

Conducting Preliminary and Clinical Assessments in Telemental Health

Rosanne Nunnery and Ann Melvin

Nothing is impossible. The word itself says 'I'm Possible.'

–Audrey Hepburn, actress and humanitarian

Learning Objectives

After reading this chapter, you should be able to do the following:

1. Describe the role of assessment in telemental health
2. Identify preliminary screening assessments, including crisis, commonly used in telemental health
3. Discuss strategies for delivering clinical assessments in telemental health

Introduction

The word *assessment* can conjure the idea of dreaded final exams for courses and national exams for licensure. However, assessment has been around since approximately 2200 BC, when Chinese culture implemented a form of testing to evaluate and promote workers. This progressed across history to examine career, intelligence, physical wellness, aptitude, achievement, and so forth

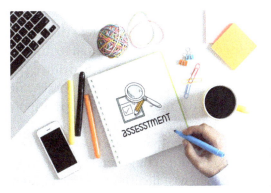

(Hays, 2017). When working with clients seeking mental health treatment, the assessment process begins from the very first call or online communication from a client to a counselor. Virtual settings often have information forms online for potential clients to complete to notify their prospective counselor of presenting concerns. This is completed online and submitted electronically to be delivered to the counselor for review. Thus begins the first contact with the client and the assessment process. It is crucial to collect client information initially to determine their reason for seeking counseling and during intake and early sessions to inform their diagnosis and develop a treatment plan that meets their needs.

As a result of COVID-19, the field of counseling has been transformed. The support for distance counseling has gained considerable momentum as empirical evidence continues to show its efficacy (Wright & Raiford, 2021). That said, regardless of the treatment platform, the screening and assessment process is a significant component of clinical mental health treatment. The American Counseling Association's (ACA) ethical guidelines indicate that mental health treatment can be delivered beyond in person to extend to distant formats. However, there is reiteration regarding the need for proper assessment (ACA, 2014). As telemental health becomes increasingly utilized, we must adapt to meet alternative platforms' clinical, ethical, and legal standards. Many screening and assessment tools have evolved to meet the changes in counseling delivery (Luxton et al., 2016). Counselors need to be savvy in locating assessments that can be adapted in a telemental health setting. This chapter will explore preliminary assessments, including screening and intake forms, crisis protocols, and clinical assessments to serve clientele in telemental health practice.

The Role of Assessment in Telemental Health

Diagnosis and treatment of mental health disorders are facilitated through accurate screening and assessment tools (Hunsley & Mash, 2020). Assessment is the start of the golden thread. The term *golden* is used because documentation should flow logically from one piece to another for those reviewing the record (Contra Costa Behavioral Health, 2021). Documentation of the findings from assessment, including the mental health symptoms severe enough to disrupt the client's ability to function in all areas of their lives, should be identified during the assessment process. A formal assessment assists in diagnosing possible mental health disorders for a client and confirms measures of the diagnosis severity. Furthermore, the tools assess the client's strengths and resources to meet life's challenges.

Using a preliminary screen, we collect client information to determine their reason for seeking counseling, determining proper diagnosis, and developing a treatment plan. Telemental health will take it a step further so that you can determine if the client and their diagnosis are appropriate to treat in a distance format. The telemental health process can utilize online screening and assessment tools that allow the counselor to collect the client's information through a secure platform. As part of the preliminary assessment process, the client should be evaluated for accessibility to appropriate technical resources, privacy concerns, and overall suitability for telemental health. Ramirez et al. (2020) concur that telehealth requires adjusting to the assessment process. Several senses are restricted when a clinician works remotely. Consider, for instance, the use of a mental status exam (MSE) and the need to be creative in order to avoid omitting aspects of an in-person evaluation. It is needed to monitor client tone, word usage, and content of what is being said very carefully. More challenging is the assessment of the client's mobility and appearance, and counselors may resort to asking the client to walk across the room while the camera is turned on (Ramirez et al., 2020). It is helpful to outline the typical flow of assessments used when beginning a telemental health relationship with a client. Typically, we would start off with preliminary assessments.

Preliminary Assessments

What comes to mind when you think about a preliminary assessment? Typically, we think of informed consent, an intake or biopsychosocial assessment, or other clinical assessments. Diagnosis and treatment of mental health disorders are facilitated through accurate screening and assessment tools (Hunsley & Mash, 2020). Initial screening and assessment also include a suicide risk assessment, problem identification, and intervention strategies (Hays, 2017). Screening and assessment tools serve a purpose in the holistic treatment process. The telemental health process utilizes online screening and assessment tools that allow the counselor to collect the client's information through a secure platform. Our clients need to be able to manage the necessary technology, ensure a confidential space for sessions, and collaborate in crisis planning and management (Ramirez et al., 2020). The client's location, state laws, and unique circumstances may play a significant role in determining whether technology is appropriate (Luxton et al., 2016). Let's explore the types of preliminary assessments commonly used.

Client Screening for Telemental Health

The telemental health preliminary screening begins by determining if an online platform is appropriate for the client. It is an ethical requirement that clients are screened before engaging in telemental health (National Board for Certified Counselors [NBCC], 2016). We need to recognize that not all clients are candidates for telehealth services. First it is important to provide a screening by asking clients specific questions (e.g., presenting problems, mental health status, suicidal ideation, etc.) After reviewing the answers to these questions, the counselor will need to review some additional questions based on how the initial questions are answered. By prescreening clients with specific questions (e.g., technology, crisis, unique circumstances), counselors are positioned to determine if telemental health is appropriate. Screening tools are brief and help establish a baseline of the client's case. Screening for mental health disorders should include screening for the risk of self-harm and suicide, whether that treatment occurs in person or virtually (Luxton et al., 2016). The initial online screening tool includes questions regarding suitability for an online counseling platform.

A screening tool collects initial information but does not typically collect enough information to diagnose and develop a treatment plan. Oftentimes, clients will enter a digital relationship with a counselor by scrolling through the varied telemental health providers via their insurance or by choosing a self-pay system where the counselor's profile can be reviewed. Once the client selects a clinician, they are often prompted to complete some preliminary questions to help the counselor have a broad understanding of why the client is in need of assistance. The information will be a tool to use prior to completing an intake/biopsychosocial assessment. While some screening tools focus on specific conditions, such as depression or substance abuse, others collect symptoms associated with a range of mental health concerns. While there is no standard prescreening form that you should use, you will likely be given one specific to your fieldwork placement/site. Following are essential areas you should assess as part of your first telemental health screening process prior to asking some follow-up questions.

SCREENING QUESTIONS

What is your age?

What is your preferred language?

Do you consider yourself to be religious or spiritual? Please identify.

Are you currently employed?

What brings you to seeking telemental health counseling?

What are your thoughts about using a digital platform for counseling?

How difficult are the presenting problems you identified for you to do your work, take care of things at home, or get along with other people?

What type of counseling are you looking for?

Have you ever been to counseling before?

What gender were you born? To what gender do you identify?

What is your romantic orientation?

What is your relationship status?

Do you have any problems or worries about intimacy?

Do you have any concerns of safety in your intimate relationship?

How is your present interest or pleasure in doing things on a daily basis?

Do you move or speak so slowly that other people could have noticed? Or the opposite—are you so fidgety or restless that you have been moving around a lot more than usual?

Are you feeling down or depressed, or do you a sense of hopelessness?

Do you have trouble falling asleep, staying asleep, or sleeping too much?

Are you noticing that you are feeling tired of having little energy?

Are you noticing poor appetite or overeating?

How would you rate your current eating habits on a scale of 1–10, with 10 being the absolute best eating habits?

How would you rate your current physical health on a scale of 1–10, with10 being the absolute best physically?

Are you currently taking any medication?

Are you currently experiencing any chronic pain?

Are you feeling bad about yourself or that you are a failure of having let yourself or your family down?

Do you have trouble concentrating on things, such as reading the newspaper or watching television?

Have you had any thoughts that you would be better off dead or of have you thought of killing yourself in some way? If you have, when was the last time you thought about this?

Who have you told about your feelings about death, dying, and killing yourself?

Are you willing to list an emergency contact person who is easily accessible?

Are you currently experiencing overwhelming sadness, grief, or depression?

Are you currently experiencing any anxiety or panic attacks, or do you have any phobias?

How do you prefer to communicate with your counselor? Please specify if you prefer video, chat, phone, or messenger. The first session must be by video.

Once you have reviewed the answers to these questions, it is important to take a moment to complete a suitability for telemental health counseling checklist and then ask follow-up questions prior to asking the client to confirm the informed consent document to begin the counseling process. Following are a few questions to consider asking yourself; once you have answered your portion, it will be imperative to directly ask your client some follow-up questions.

ONLINE TELEMENTAL HEALTH SUITABILITY CHECKLIST

Client name:

Age:

Date:

Please review the screening question to determine the level of client risk. Circle YES or NO if a risk is identified. If a risk is noted, follow-up questions to the client are required.

Is the client suicidal, or do they have a significant risk of becoming so? YES/NO

Is the client homicidal, or do they have a significant risk of becoming so? YES/NO

Does the client have delusions about technology/electronics or have a significant risk of developing them? YES/NO

Is the counselor competent in addressing the client's needs/goals via telemental health services? YES/NO

Is the client in a current domestic abuse situation? YES/NO

Have the risks of telemental health services in domestic abuse situations and the options of in-person counseling been discussed with the potential client? YES/NO

Has it been determined that telemental health counseling is an appropriate option for the client? YES/NO

Ask these follow-up questions after you have screened for risk:

Questions to ask the client:

Is the client willing to remove all firearms from the home? YES/NO

Is the client willing to identify an appropriate support person? YES/NO

Support Person's Name:

Relationship to Client:

Phone Number(s):

Physical Address:

When using video conferencing, texting, chat, or email:

If using chat, texting, or email: Are you willing to have an initial session in person or via video-conferencing in order to verify your identity? YES/NO

Do you have a computer/device with internet access and that has the capability of using (name of videoconferencing, texting, chat, or email technology)? YES/NO

Do you have a location to receive telemental counseling in a location that allows for confidentiality? YES/NO

Are you comfortable with using videoconferencing, chat, or email as a means for receiving counseling? YES/NO

I use (name of videoconferencing, texting, chat, or email technology) for online counseling. It requires (e.g., setting up an account, downloading the program, cost). Are you comfortable with trying to use this technology? YES/NO

There is a potential for technology breakdowns and interruptions. Do you believe the use of technology will cause you more distress than it will help you? YES/NO

Do you have an alternate form of communication if the platform we are using fails? For example, if we are on a video call and the internet goes out, can I reach you by phone? YES/NO

Informed Consent

Once the preliminary screening and suitability checklist has been completed, it is imperative that before the first session you make sure your client reviews the telemental health informed consent document. The ACA (2014) code of ethics and NBCC (2014) code of ethics reinforce that there is an informed consent specific to telemental health practice. When I (Rosanne) first started my work as a telemental health practitioner, I had to look closely at the similarities and differences between a typical in-person and telemental health informed consent, and they are slightly different. Although there are varied ways to approach the writing of a telemental health informed consent, let's look at some specific areas that need to be addressed in an informed consent. Of course, with you being a counselor-in-training, remember to note who your supervisor is and how you are being monitored. As you review the areas that are addressed, consider what you have seen before and what else you might like to include.

TELEMENTAL HEALTH INFORMED CONSENT AGREEMENT FOR COUNSELING SERVICES

Name, educational credentials, telemental health credentials, contact information, location of services

Name of clinical supervisor, supervisor's credentials, contact information, and location of supervision

Clinical training in graduate school

Professional services and what telemental health platform they are offered

Therapeutic approach

The process of therapy and evaluation; include risks and benefits of telemental health, possible side effects, problems with technology and technology failure, and alternative methods of service delivery

Anticipated response time

Telephone and emergency procedures when counselor is not available or if a crisis arrives for the client

Privacy and confidentiality, including limits to confidentiality

Reinforcement of openness to culture, religion, language, orientation, and other cultural factors with no imposition of values by the counselor

Discussion of treatment planning

Process of termination, referrals, and testing

Dual relationships, including social media policy

Electronic record keeping and online encryption of correspondence

Billing procedures and releases of information for third parties

Consultation policy specific to supervisor and outside consultants

Payments, fees, cancellations

Ethics adhered to, school or licensure board information, and prompt for signature

Intake and Biopsychosocial Assessments

Once the client has reviewed and signed the informed consent, it is time to set an appointment for the first synchronous video session to establish a relationship with the client and gather more information. The intake, also called the clinical interview or biopsychosocial assessment, is crucial for the assessment process (Wright et al., 2020). A skillful interview allows you to observe behavior, understand a person's characteristics, and uncover information that would otherwise be difficult to obtain. An intake/biopsychosocial assessment is a critical part of the initial assessment process when first meeting a client, whether in person or in a telemental health setting. The biopsychosocial assessment/intake will look different when working with an adult or child.

Many clinicians choose to conduct a mental status examination as part of the assessment that measures behavior and cognition. Clinically significant cognitive characteristics are alertness, language, memory, and the ability to construct and reason abstractly. When evaluating the client's mood and identifying high-risk behaviors associated with emotional distress, nonverbal information can be helpful (Luxton et al., 2016). Therefore, we need to find the most appropriate ways to observe nonverbal information online. Adequate bandwidth and resolution are necessary for the mental status examination to detect signs of behavioral disturbance, changes in appearance, or other related observations (The Telemental Health Examination [TMHE], 2022).

BIOPSYCHOSOCIAL ASSESSMENT FORM

Client Demographic Data

Name:_____ DOB: _____ Age:_____

Gender: Client was born M/F and client identifies as M/F

Parent/Legal Guardian/Responsible Party _____

Social-Cultural Information (race, ethnicity, religion, sexual orientation, romantic orientation, etc.)

_____

_____

Presenting Issues

_____

_____

History of Presenting Problems

_____

_____

Education and Occupation

School/Grade currently attending (if applicable):_____ Grade:_____

Educational History (including learning problems, school issues, academics, social)

_____

_____

Highest grade completed: _____

Occupation and employment history (present and past, years worked, reasons for periods of unemployment):

_____

_____

Occupational Skills/Training

_____

_____

Military Background: _____

Current Living Situation and Environment

Housing: What type of housing and who lives in the current household? _____

_____

Social Connections: _____

Financial Situation: _____

Other considerations (legal, guardianship, transportation, limitations, etc.):_____

_____

Personal Medical History

List of hospitalizations for any medical reason (illness, operation, accidents, etc.):

Reason for Hospitalization	Date	How Long?

Medical Conditions:

Name of Medical Condition	Date Diagnosed	Treatment

Current Medications:

Name of Medication	Dosage	For What Reason?	How Long?	Side Effects?

Substance Use (list current or past with any of the following:

	Yes/No	Frequency of Use		Yes/No	Frequency of Use
Alcohol			Inhalants		

Barbiturates			Marijuana		
Caffeine			Methadone		
Cocaine			Methamphet-amines		
Opiates			Stimulants		
Hallucino-gens			Tobacco		
Sedatives			Tranquilizers		
Other			Other		

Emotional and Psychiatric History (list past mental health care including psychiatrists, psychologists, social work, and counseling):

Provider (Name, Address, Phone Number)	Reason for Treatment	Type of Treatment	Dates

Current Symptoms/ Problems:

Rate severity and duration for each problem listed in the table using the following scale:

Severity: 1 = Mild; 2 = Moderate; 3 = Severe

Duration: 1 = > 1 month; 2 = 1-12 months; 3 = < 1 year

Problem	Severity	Duration	Problem	Severity	Duration
Anxiety			Family problems		

Panic attacks				Sleep disturbance		
Phobia				Paranoid ideation		
OCD				Gender issues		
Somatization				Eating disorders		
Depression				Loss of energy		
Impaired memory				Conduct problems		
Poor self-care skills				School problems		
Loss of interest				Sexual dysfunction		
Suicidal ideation/ attempts				Other		

Client's Strengths: _____

_____

Other information (observed by counselor):_____

_____

Describe potential follow-up assessments needed (suicidal/crisis/alcohol):

_____

_____

Describe potential consultations/referrals/release of information needed to professionals:

_____

Treatment Planning:

Identified Problems	Long-Term Goals (e.g., 6, 9, 12 Months)	Short-Term Objectives (e.g., 1 Week up to 3 Months)	Interventions

Following are some general components of a mental status exam and what you will typically assess.

GENERIC MENTAL STATUS EXAM COMPONENTS

1. Appearance: Observing a client's appearance while on screen including grooming, clothes, posture, gait, nails, etc.
2. Behavior/psychomotor activity: Mannerisms, gestures, eye contact, facial expressions, psychomotor activity, body language, tone of voice, rapport.
3. Attitude toward examiner: Reflecting on client response toward you and/or other clinical participants in the virtual meeting.
4. Affect (emotional quality and range) and mood: Anxious, worried, depressed with consideration of flat affect, sad, agitated, euphoric, restricted, labile. Some useful descriptors might include intensity, quality, fluctuation, range and congruence.
5. Speech and thought: Rate and flow, quantity, tone, fluency, rhythm, route.
6. Perceptual disturbances: Thoughts (stream of thought, form of thought, content of thought). Thoughts might include flight of ideas, derailed thinking, muted, obsessive thoughts, ruminating thoughts, delusions; review of perceptual abnormalities such as hallucinations, difficulty concentrating, how the client responds to stimuli, and awareness of sense of self.
7. Orientation and consciousness: Consideration of date, time, place, current setting, asking about current president, time of day, year, season, and so forth.
8. Memory and intelligence: The client is given objects to remember and repeat back to the counselor once the list is completed.
9. Reliability, judgment, and insight: The client's understanding of their mental health problem from your completion of the assessment and follow-up questions. Consider if there is insight, judgment, acceptance, or denial.

Clinical Assessments

After conducting the preliminary assessments, you will often have additional questions lingering in your mind regarding symptoms noted by the client and signs you have observed. When this happens, additional assessments may be necessary to narrow down the diagnostic focus for effective treatment planning. Performing initial assessments provides a comprehensive clinical perspective, determines medical necessity, and helps us develop appropriate treatment plans in collaboration with the client. Ramirez et al. (2020) remind us that during a telemental health assessment clients' privacy and confidentiality must be protected as if the service were being provided in person. During the client's first contact, you can utilize section III of the Diagnostic and Statistical Manual, fifth edition (DSM-5; American Psychiatric Association, 2013). The emerging measures offered in Section III of the DSM-5 are used in client prescreening to help determine the severity of symptoms and further assessment options (American Psychiatric Association, 2013). These are commonly public assessments that do not require a fee for use and are easily accessible.

Prior to administering any assessment, we must have solid foundational skills to create and build on the counselor–client relationship. Building a therapeutic relationship between the client and the provider begins at the beginning of treatment, which typically involves some form of preliminary assessment (Hays, 2017). Think about the importance of building a therapeutic relationship so that the client feels comfortable sharing personal information. Creating a safe and trusting environment is the number-one priority. It may seem simple in the comfort of your office, but how can you ensure the same through any platform? Disclosure and honesty can be challenging regardless of whom you tell, the physical setting, or the circumstances. Once the relationship is established, we have access to many different assessment and screening tool options to help screen and diagnose mental health disorders (Newson et al., 2020). However, we must also consider the required training for each tool, accessibility (public or copyright), and assessment selection and use in telemental health. It is important that we explore each of these components prior to choosing a subsequent assessment for a client. Let's break them down.

Training/Requirements

Counselors need to consider whether they are qualified to use the assessment and the instrument's availability. Choosing appropriate assessment and screening tools requires training and clinical judgment. Each state has varied rules regarding the required training for conducting assessments, so make sure to check your state law regarding if your credentials are sufficient to conduct assessments. Another factor, even if your state allows for you to assess, is the training and practice you have with an assessment. Prior to conducting an assessment, make sure that you have been exposed to the assessment before, have been supervised to score and interpret it, and if specific training is required to administer the assessment, make sure that it is complete. I (Rosanne) remember my first time going online and trying to purchase an assessment for use in my telemental health practice. Before I could purchase one, the company required a copy of my license and transcript showing I had completed a specific class to prove I was competent to administer it. Of course, some assessments do not require that additional level of training, but it is wise to always review the requirement for each assessment. Of course, while you are an intern, it is your clinical supervisor who will need to ensure that they have the appropriate qualifications as well. Following our professional code of ethics applies to assessment and screening tools. The ACA (2014) code of ethics states:

Counselors use only those testing and assessment services for which they have been trained and are competent. Counselors using technology-assisted test interpretations are trained in the construct being measured and the specific instrument being used prior to using its technology-based application. Counselors take reasonable measures to ensure the proper use of assessment techniques by persons under their supervision. (p. 11)

Accessibility

The accessibility and completion of assessments can look different when conducting counseling via telemental health. It is important to consider not only the training but the cost, accessibility to the digital format, and delivery of results. As an assessment instructor, I (Rosanne) typically have a final assignment that requires students to choose an assessment and investigate it thoroughly. What I find is often overlooked is the tiny stamp on an assessment that says copyright or public access. Why is this important? If an assessment has a copyright, and most do, there is a specific requirement the assessment creator has that is attached to that copyright. Some of the stipulations might include training, permission to reproduce, a one-time fee for the manual or software, a fee for each assessment that will be needed, requirement that the developer scores it via their software, or it could be as simple as a requirement to ask permission for the assessment. If the requirements are not followed, you could be violating not only the law but ethics as well. How do you avoid a problem? The answer is simple: Look at the manual and at the bottom of the assessment and see what the copyright indicates. What if it says public access? If it says public access, you still want to look and see if the assessment developer requires permission for use. For example, the DSM-5 (American Psychological Association, 2013) assessments are considered public use for the clinician. If there are no stipulations, they can be used with clients as clinical tools without paying. Diving a bit deeper, if you have to pay for an assessment, does a client have to as well? If you are paying high fees for assessments, the cost will likely trickle down to the client as part of the billing services. If it is free to you via public access, you need to make an ethical decision regarding if you will bill for your time to administer, score, and interpret the test and results. This is where your supervisor will be very helpful to you.

Assessment Selection and Use in Telemental Health

You now know that training is an integral part of the assessment process, along with varied stipulations regarding accessibility of assessments due to fees and copyright. Now we will explore assessment selection and use in a telemental health setting. Clients are often very accustomed to completing an initial screening and biopsychosocial assessment, but they often do not consider that after those are complete there might be a need for a clinical assessment. This is where your clinical skills come in handy. Just as you explained the preliminary assessment process and how the information will be utilized in treatment, you want to let them know that a clinical assessment is needed due to the symptoms the client explored and the signs you noticed after completion of the biopsychosocial assessment. For example, "I noticed as we talked through the varied questions in the biopsychosocial assessments that you have struggled with depression since you were a teenager. You noted many highs and lows but always felt as if depression was looming over you. As a result, I do think it would be beneficial for you to complete a clinical assessment evaluating your depression. What are your thoughts surrounding delving deeper into your depression?" We do need to remember that we should be collaborative with assessments and treatment planning and that there is informed consent regarding assessments (ACA, 2014). Clinical assessments have a wide variety of ranges that may include but are not limited to anxiety, depression, behavorial concerns, alcohol or drug use, personality characteristics, attention deficit disorder, communication, attachment, and so forth. The choice of a follow-up assessment in telemental health will depend on client need along with the availability of the measure to be accessible in a digital format. Some assessment companies have quick links to complete assessments online, while others might only have paper and pencil availability, which might influence your decision to use that specific assessment with a client. It is not uncommon for many assessments to be converted to a PDF version for ease of access and delivery via email, message, or link. Some companies allow the client to sign in on a website, pay a fee, and complete the assessment, and the company will score it and send the results to

VOICES FROM THE FIELD

What has been your experience with delivering assessments in a telemental health setting?

"The process is similar to in-person; however, I am even more intentional about displaying empathy. The assessment process can be daunting and impersonal to many clients—almost feeling like an interrogation. Being mindful of this, I do everything possible to ease the process by being warm, empathic, and adjusting to the client. Where applicable, using the whiteboard feature can help with posting questions, responses, and other relevant information."

-Matt Glowiak, PhD, LCPC, CAADC, NCC, Bolingbrook, IL

"When used, I often email them and we go over them together during sessions."

-Melissa Lee-Tammeus, PhD, LMHC, Jacksonville, FL

"I have found that use of a Biopsychosocial Assessment or other assessment measurement tools remains effective in telemental health."

-David Hart, PhD, LPC, NCC, CTMH, St. Louis, MO

the client. It is your responsibility to investigate these options prior to getting a client to take an assessment. Of course, some assessments such as the telemental health screener, biopsychosocial assessment, mental status exam, and treatment plan, can all be developed by you and easily accessed via your telemental health platform. Once you have corresponded with a specific company, you will know what type of access you will have. Consider what questions you might ask a company about the use of assessment in a telemental health setting. What happens if you suspect a client might be in the midst of a crisis?

Crisis Assessment

Nearly 40% of clients in telemental health admit that they have recently thought about suicide (Tarlow et al., 2018). Suicide assessments have become standard practice at every telemental health or face-to-face session. A suicide assessment includes examining the client's plan, intent, means, prior attempts, and substance abuse. We use suicide assessments to determine what can be done for the client to remain safe in the event of a mental health crisis. Suicide risk can be reduced in part by the information we gather during the initial assessment and then with a follow-up clinical or crisis assessment. If you have higher-risk clients who fail to attend an appointment, the broader procedures may need to be modified to accommodate their absences. You should develop a protocol for when your clients can't attend a therapy session virtually and for those newly on your radar for possible suicide risk. As we proceed, we will explore the importance of proactive planning and documentation with clients whom you determine at risk for suicide.

Proactive Planning

Clinical approaches for a client in telemental health counseling are similar to in-person counseling (James & Gilliland, 2020). Being mindful of clinical, ethical, and legal concerns is necessary when selecting and administering suicide assessments. As noted earlier in this chapter, you should screen your clients for crisis, whether it be domestic violence, suicidal thoughts, past suicidal attempts, paranoia toward technology, or even homicidal ideation. The preliminary screening and suitability for telemental health will provide a clearer vision of whether this client is a fit for telemental health. If you made the decision that the client is a good fit, the next level that will be helpful is the biopsychosocial assessment. Even with these gatekeeping measures, you might have a client who suddenly has a crisis emerge, which might lead to you considering an additional assessment. Prior to this emergence, make sure you have demographic information on the client and an emergency contact, and that the informed consent elements of limits to confidentiality are documented.

Once you see that a crisis is evident, it is time to consider what you need to assess. A common need for clients is a suicide assessment. There are many public domain suicide assessments available for use. Examples include but are not limited to the Patient Health Questionnaire (PHQ-9), the Suicide Assessment Five-Step Evaluation and Triage (SAFE-T), and the Ask Suicide Screening Questionnaire (ASQ; National Institute of Mental Health, 2020). The Columbia Lighthouse Project (CLP, 2021) developed the Columbia Suicide Severity Rating Scale (C-SSRS), which is appropriate for telemental health. The scale can be translated into more than 150 languages and implemented in many settings, including schools, hospitals, college campuses, defense forces, fire departments, the justice system, primary care, and scientific research (CLP, 2021). Back in early 2000 (Godleski et al., 2008) the Veteran Health Administration (VHA) began utilizing a telemental health modality and campaign for suicide prevention and intervention. The research outcomes showed that suicide risk assessments in a telemental health setting were just as effective as in a face-to face in person setting. As a result of this research, the VHA has established the following recommendations for telemental health and suicide assessments (U.S. Department of Veterans Affairs & U.S. Department of Defense, 2019):

- Verify the person's location (e.g., address, apartment number) at the start of the session if you need to contact emergency services.
- If the platform you are using is not HIPAA compliant, the client must verbally consent.
- Document the client's verbal consent in their notes and take the next step by getting written permission from them.
- Get emergency contact information and make sure you have verbal consent to be contacted in case of an emergency.
- Ensure you have a backup plan if the technology does not work, such as having the best number to reach your client.
- Before contact, develop a plan for staying on the phone with the client while arranging emergency rescue if needed.
- Establish a protocol for calling 911 or a crisis outreach team while staying connected with your client.

Crisis Intervention

What are the next steps if the suicidal assessment indicates a high risk? Let's consider the code of ethics, laws in our state, and the process of protecting clients or their acquaintances. The National Conference of State Legislator's (2022) website provides confidentiality laws for each state. Knowledge of the ethics and state laws will help when we select or develop a crisis response plan. Examples of current crisis intervention models include ABCD Crisis Intervention, Critical Incident Stress Management

(CISM), NOVA Crisis Intervention, and Psychological First Aid (PFA). The safety planning process includes but is not limited to the following:

- Develop a safety plan in collaboration with the client.
- Provide the client a copy of the safety plan.
- Provide crisis line and text information.
- Increase contact with the client as needed.
- Conduct follow-up assessment at every session for clients at elevated risk.

VOICES FROM THE FIELD

How have you navigated crises within a telemental health setting?

"I set the ground rules for telemental health counseling with the client. If the client is high risk I have them sign a release form so I can contact the client's family member or friend. If there appears to be an emergency, I will call 911 while staying on the video with the client."

–Cheryl Welch, PhD, LPC, RN, Florence, WI

"I collaborate with other colleagues and doctors. For instance, I recently had a teen client who threatened to harm herself and I worked with her psychiatrist and a local residential center, along with her parents to have her admitted. Through phone calls, all of this was done in a day and the client was able to be placed in a secure center quite quickly."

–Melissa Lee-Tammeus, PhD, LMHC, Jacksonville, FL

"This process had to be a thoughtful one. With general safety plans in place, we needed to be even more diligent with their implementation. It was also important to adjust informed consent to meet the more specific needs of a technology-based platform. Being that clients continued to be within the area, we were knowledgeable of emergency resources and providers."

–Matt Glowiak, PhD, LCPC, CAADC, NCC, Bolingbrook, IL

Cultural Considerations

The U.S. population continues to diversify, which presents both challenges and opportunities in mental health care and when considering assessments that are aligned to individuals' diverse perspectives. When we have limited knowledge of a culture, we can make assumptions and overgeneralize about specific cultures when we should take into account the individual person we are serving (Hays, 2017). We need to remember that there are ethical guidelines to cultural awareness in treatment, which includes selection, use, and interpretation of assessments (ACA, 2014). As counselors, we are required to consider the importance of our fairness with assessments and acknowledge our own cultural bias. There are many assessments that are emerging specific to culturally diverse populations (Paniagua, 2014), and thus we must investigate assessments that are a good fit for the individual clients served.

The concept of culturally appropriate care is not universally defined, but telemental health experts have defined it as "the delivery of mental health services that are guided by the cultural concerns of all racial or ethnic groups, including psychosocial background, typical styles of symptom presentation, immigration histories, and other cultural traditions, beliefs, and values" (Brooks et al., 2013, p. 63). Keeping the cultural dimensions of the professional relationship in mind is crucial. Luxton et al. (2016) report several other significant elements of telemental health, including an assessment of the impact of culture on our client's "(a) overall comfort/socialization with the behavioral health system; (b) comfort and familiarity with the technology; (c) communication, rapport, and trust; and (d) perceptions of confidentiality" (p. 111). We should also be aware of how our culture, values, and biases toward technology influence telemental health.

Clinical Supervision Considerations

As a counselor-in-training, you will be under supervision during your practicum and internship and as you pursue your license post-graduation. Many practicum and internship locations began offering telemental health sessions and telemental health supervision prior to, during, and post-pandemic restrictions. In fact, due to location limitations for specific supervisors, the use of technology for supervision has been an asset to complete the required hours for many future licensed professionals. Modern technology allows us to conduct clinical supervision virtually (Martin et al., 2017). As part of counselors' continuing professional development, clinical supervision is essential. Research has found that supervisees and supervisors prepare more diligently for telesupervision and disclose more because they feel secure in the distance relationship (Rousmaniere et al., 2014). Many of the techniques used to build rapport with a client also transfer to the supervisory relationship. Supervisory approaches for telemental health counseling can include a variety of approaches based on traditional clinical supervision. You can meet with your supervisor in person or remotely. Synchronous telemental health counseling is also an option, which involves a supervisor observing a supervisee as they provide counseling, including assessment to a client online (Machuca & Kums, 2021). Martin et al. (2017) outline evidence-informed, practical tips to help guide the supervisory relationship.

Chapter Summary

A significant part of clinical mental health treatment is screening and assessment. This chapter focused on the importance of screening and assessment related to telemental health counseling. A formal assessment assists in diagnosing possible mental disorders and confirming measures of severity of those disorders; a formal assessment aids in establishing a client's mental health status. Additionally, the tools assess the client's strengths and resources for coping with life's challenges. With telemental health, a counselor can access client information through a secure online platform that provides screening and assessment tools. Prior to telemental health enrollment, a preliminary assessment should assess whether the client has appropriate technical resources, privacy concerns, and overall suitability. An online assessment tool can be used as part of the telemental health process to provide the counselor with the client's information via a secure platform. Attention to state laws, the client's location, and the case's unique circumstances are critical in telemental health counseling (Luxton et al., 2016). Supervisory approaches for telemental health counseling can include a variety of approaches based on traditional clinical supervision. Telemental health is becoming increasingly popular, and we must adapt to meet alternative platforms' clinical, ethical, and legal standards.

APPLICATION ACTIVITY

Case Example

Marie calls your office to say she needs to talk to someone right away, but she prefers not to discuss anything in person, and she only has a short amount of time to talk. Marie's voice is soft, almost a whisper. She sounds like she might be crying, but you cannot be sure without video. Marie stated she could call back the next day. Marie calls back the next day. She says her husband will be home in 30 minutes, and you can hear children in the background. Upon speaking to Marie, you learn the following:

- *Marie reports she identifies as a Hispanic female who is 27 years old.*
- *She reports having three children under 12 years old and is currently married.*
- *Marie tells you her husband is "abusive and does not let [her] work."*
- *She says she feels "really depressed" and does not know what to do to feel better.*

Think about the main components of telemental health assessment and screening, as well as the specific attributes to consider when deciding on telemental health's appropriateness. After reviewing the varied screeners prior to meeting with a client, consider how you will need to handle this case. Describe the additional information you will need to determine if the client is a good candidate for telemental health and how you might obtain the necessary information.

References

American Counseling Association (2014). *ACA code of ethics.* Author. https://www.counseling. org/docs/default-source/default-document-library/2014-code-of-ethics-finaladdress.pdf

American Psychiatric Association. (2013). *Diagnostic and statistical manual of mental disorders* (5th ed.). Author. https://doi.org/10.1176/appi.books.9780890425596

Brooks, E., Spargo, G., Yellowlees, P., O'Neil, P., & Shore, J. H. (2013). Integrating culturally appropriate care into telemental health practice. In K. Myers & C. L. Turvey (Eds.), *Telemental health: Clinical, technical, and administrative foundations for evidence-based practice* (pp. 63–82). Elsevier.

Chiauzzi, E., Clayton, A., & Huh-Yoo, J. (2020). Videoconferencing-based telemental health: Important questions for the COVID-19 era from clinical and patient-centered perspectives. *JMIR Mental Health, 7*(12), e24021–e24021. https://doi.org/10.2196/24021

Contra Costa County Behavioral Health. (2021, June). *Clinical documentation guide.* https://cchealth. org/mentalhealth/clinical-documentation/pdf/Clinical-Documentation-Manual.pdf

Godleski, L., Nieves, J. E., Darkins, A., & Lehmann, L. (2008). VA telemental health: Suicide assessment. *Behavioral Sciences & the Law, 26*(3), 271–286. https://doi.org/10.1002/bsl.811

Hays, D. (2017). *Assessment in counseling: A guide to use of psychological assessment procedures* (6th edition). American Counseling Association.

Hunsley, J., & Mash, E. J. (2020). The role of assessment in evidence-based practice. In M. M. Antony & D. H. Barlow (Eds.), *Handbook of assessment and treatment planning for psychological disorders* (pp. 3–23). Guilford Press.

James, R. K., & Gilliland, B. E. (2020). *Crisis intervention strategies* (8th ed.). Cengage.

Luxton, D., Nelson, E. L., & Maheu, M. M. (2016). *A practitioner's guide to telemental health: How to conduct legal, ethical, and evidence-based telepractice.* American Psychological Association.

Machuca, R., & Kums, A. (2021). The virtual bug: Online live supervision of telemental health counseling. *Journal of Technology in Counselor Education and Supervision, 1*(1), 19–26. https://doi. org/10.22371/tces/003

Martin, P., Kumar, S., & Lizarondo, L. (2017). Effective use of technology in clinical supervision. *Internet Interventions: The Application of Information Technology in Mental and Behavioural Health, 8*(C), 35–39. https://doi.org/10.1016/j.invent.2017.03.001

National Board for Certified Counselors. (2016). *NBCC code of ethics.* Author.

National Conference of State Legislators. (2022, March 16). *Mental health professionals' duty to warn.* https://www.ncsl.org/research/health/mental-health-professionals-duty-to-warn.aspx

National Institute of Mental Health. (2020, July 1). *ASQ Suicide Risk Screening Tool.* https:// www.nimh.nih.gov/sites/default/files/documents/research/research-conducted-at-nimh/ asq-toolkit-materials/asq-tool/screening_tool_asq_nimh_toolkit.pdf

Newson, J. J., Hunter, D., & Thiagarajan, T. C. (2020). The heterogeneity of mental health assessment. *Frontiers in Psychiatry, 11*, 76. https://doi.org/10.3389/fpsyt.2020.00076

Paniagua, F. A. (2014). *Assessing and treating culturally diverse clients: A practice guide* (4th ed.). SAGE.

Ramirez, H., Springmeyer, A., Weis, K., Espiritu, R., Wolf-Prusan, L., DeCelle, K., Heitkamp, T., & Clarke, B. L. (2020). *Telehealth clinical and technical considerations for mental health providers.* Pacific Southwest Mental Health Technology Transfer Center. https://cars-rp.org/_MHTTC/docs/Telehealth%20Clinical%20Considerations.pdf

Rousmaniere, T., Abbass, A., & Frederickson, J. (2014). New developments in technology-assisted supervision and training: A practical overview. *Journal of Clinical Psychology, 70*(11), 1082–1093. https://doi.org/10.1002/jclp.22129

Tarlow, K. R., Johnson, T. A., & McCord, C. E. (2018). Rural status, suicide ideation, and telemental health: Risk assessment in a clinical sample. *The Journal of Rural Health, 35*(2), 247–252. https://doi.org/10.1111/jrh.12310

The Columbia Lighthouse Project. (n.d.). *About the protocol.* https://cssrs.columbia.edu/the-columbia-scale-c-ssrs/about-the-scale/

The Telemental Health Examination. (n.d.). *Center for Credentialing and Education.* https://cce-global.org/assets/bctmh/tmhe_content_outline.pdf

U.S. Department of Veterans Affairs & U.S. Department of Defense. (2019). *VA/DoD clinical practice guideline for the assessment and management of patients at risk for suicide.* https://www.healthquality.va.gov/guidelines/MH/srb/VADoDSuicideRiskFullCPGFinal5088212019.pdf

Wright, J. A., Mihura, J. L., & McCord, D. M. (2020, April 3). *Guidance on psychological tele-assessment during the COVID-19 crisis.* American Psychologcial Association. http://www.apaservices.org/practice/reimbursement/health-codes/testing/tele-assessment-covid-19

Wright, A. J., & Raiford, S. E. (2021). *Essentials of psychological tele-assessment.* Wiley Blackwell.

CHAPTER 5

Delivering Clinical Skills in a Telemental Health Setting

Lisa McKenna and Rosanne Nunnery

I've learned that people will forget what you said, people will forget what you did, but people will never forget how you made them feel.

–Maya Angelou

Learning Objectives

After reading this chapter, you should be able to do the following:

- Discuss how foundational counseling skills can be applied within a telemental health setting to support building and maintaining the therapeutic relationship with clients
- Explore strategies for identifying problems and setting goals with clients within a telemental health setting
- Consider application of counseling interventions and techniques in a digital setting
- Monitor therapeutic progress and referral/termination plans within a telemental health setting

Introduction

Clinical counseling skills are a building block of counseling, and application of those skills from the very beginning of the process establishes and maintains a healthy counselor–client relationship. This chapter will help you build your confidence in how these foundational counseling skills can be effectively translated into a telemental health practice. Since you are reading this text, you likely already have embraced the possibility of working within a telemental health setting. Or maybe you feel that telemental health counseling can't possibly be as effective as in-person counseling. Even though research indicates that telemental health practice performed by competent professionals is comparable to traditional in-person counseling (Hilty et al., 2017), some clinicians may have doubts. If you are in that category, we encourage you to embrace an open mind as you consider the possibilities of how you can apply all of your training in different settings. If you are feeling anxious or unconfident, and the dreaded "imposter syndrome" is creeping up its ugly head, we ask you to trust the process and continue to press forward! Many clinicians who have been independently licensed and practicing for years have been exactly where you are and made the transition with very positive outcomes for clients and themselves! How do we know this? We merely have to look at how the pandemic shifted the trajectory of work in office to work at home, which translated into an expanded clinical practice that met the needs of clients. We all were quickly pushed into a new reality and had to demonstrate cognitive flexibility to effectively adjust. You can too! Whether in the same physical location or not, our counseling skills can be effectively demonstrated visually, auditorily, and in writing.

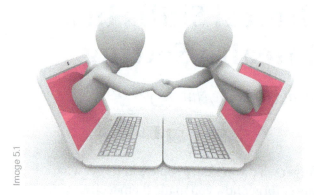

Image 5.1

In this chapter, we will use a case study (identifying information altered, of course) to discuss possibilities for application of counseling skills in a telemental health setting, including problem identification, collaborative goal setting, intervention, and supervision. Of course, with any discussion of intervention it is important to consider evaluation and planning toward termination as well. We will assume that at this point in your training you have already learned about counseling skills in your program, and that the range of experience in demonstrating your skills may be "not at all" (early in program) to "advanced" (fieldwork). That's okay; the intent here is to focus on applying the skills in a telemental health setting so that you can be prepared to utilize your training in a highly virtual world either during your training process or in your future counseling practice. We will begin each section in this chapter with a brief refresher on the topic area and then an application of the skills within a telemental health setting drawing on the case provided. Let's dig in!

VOICES FROM THE FIELD

How do you effectively maintain your foundational therapy skills across telemental health delivery methods?

"I leverage my theoretical orientation without issue and assign homework for session integration."

–Maranda Griffin, PhD, LPC, LMHC, QS-MHC, BC-TMH, practice locations in Alabama, Florida, and Michigan

"The primary way is being focused or centered on the client and their responses. This requires more effort than in-person as the non-verbal behavior is harder to read using the service type."

–Jeff McCarthy, PhD, LCPC, NCC, Ellsworth, ME

"Maintaining skills has not felt any different than in the office. I am doing the same thing in paying attention to tone of voice, facial expressions, and upper body language. I keep other distractions away from my desk, so that the client is aware that during the session they are most important."

–Kelly James, PhD, LPC, NCC, Tulsa, OK

"I purposely took a certification course in telehealth as soon as COVID hit to ensure I was privy to all ethical and legal obligations. I offer video and phone counseling but try to stay away from email and text for any counseling. I only use email and text for logistics and scheduling purposes. I make sure that I am on time to each session and that they run a total of 50 minutes. I have boundaries in place for late clients, or no shows, and am clear on all of these in the paperwork that clients must fill out before they are given a personal password to engage in telehealth session. I also continue to earn credits per my regulatory board to keep up on latest research."

– Melissa Lee-Tammeus, PhD, LMHC, Jacksonville, FL

"I only conduct sessions via Zoom/video and phone and am still able to rely on my theoretical foundation to guide sessions. Basic counseling skills such as establishment of trust and rapport, information-gathering via use of open-ended questions and assessment tools, and ongoing reassurance of confidentiality, among others, are unaffected by the telehealth format."

– David Hart, PhD, LPC, NCC, CTMH, St. Louis, MO

"I often find it interesting that there is a thought that providing telemental health services would seem to debilitate the skills received during my training. On the contrary, your skills are enhanced as you begin to pay attention to some of the subtleties of the client and the client's environment. It is as if the senses become more heightened to read the underlying

> messages on the client's presenting issues. You are able to somehow be more of yourself as well because of being in your own environment."
>
> – Alice Crawford, PhD, LCPC, Carpentersville, IL

> "Having experience as a student online helped substantially insofar as my written and oral delivery of content and expression. When the pandemic began, I did partake in an advanced telemental health training through PESI, Inc, which provided 12 CEUs. But continually reading up on the newest information provided (peer-reviewed articles), research, trainings, and engaging in each modality helps keep me consistent."
>
> – Matt Glowiak, PhD, LCPC, CAADC, NCC, Bolingbrook, IL

Building a Therapeutic Relationship Within Telemental Health Practice

It cannot be overstated that research tells us that the quality of the therapeutic relationship is more important to a successful counseling outcome than other factors such as theoretical orientation or treatment modality (Young, 2021). Therefore, we felt it essential to start our chapter on applying counseling skills with an emphasis on building the therapeutic relationship. As counselors, rarely do we support the use of overarching statements that include qualifiers such as "never" or "always" (remember your multiple-choice test-taking strategy to generally rule out responses that contain these words). Well, here we make an exception: Never not attend to the therapeutic relationship, and *always* use your counseling skills to establish and maintain a healthy relationship!

It sounds easy, and you may be saying "Of course, this would never happen to me" (and this is where the use of "never" becomes cautionary again!). How can we unintentionally get off track with focusing on the relationship? Let's look at some of the ways we've seen this happen in our experience teaching in counselor education programs for many years. Since we want to get you back on track as soon as possible we will also talk through pointers to support you in overcoming these common challenges and setting up a positive foundation to build and maintain a healthy therapeutic relationship with your clients.

Managing Apprehension

Any time we learn new skills, it is not uncommon to be nervous when the "rubber meets the road" and we are expected to demonstrate them. Add to the mix that in a training setting we are being evaluated by a professor and likely doing them in front of our fellow peers. That can be a very stressful experience! This may look different based on how you naturally cope under stress, but some signs that nerves may be getting in your way could include the following:

- *Physical symptoms*—Shallow breathing, increased heart rate, dry mouth, upset stomach, muscle tightness, headache

- *Speech*—Speaking faster, slower, more quietly, louder than normal
- *Eye contact (outside of cultural expectations)*—Excessively looking away from or staring at a client
- *Brain fog*—Difficulty processing what has been said/tracking client, and/or challenged in determining a response

The first step in managing our nerves is to proactively get ahead of them taking over. First, take a mindfulness approach and accept your nerves without judgment. Nerves are a natural and expected part of life and are a sign that you care about what you are doing and want to do a good job! I (Lisa) tell my students, if you don't feel *any* nerves trying something new, you run the risk of going in overconfident. I would much rather my students acknowledge and accept their nerves than go into a session with a potential cocky posture. With the former, students are more likely to be self-aware, tuned into the overall experience, and in an optimal posture for receiving feedback for continued growth. Second, trust that even though you are feeling the full extent of your nerves kicked into high gear, those around you likely are not. When clients come into session, they are generally in a state of high awareness of their own internal experience (both in dealing with the circumstance[s] bringing them into counseling as well as the nervousness related to opening up to someone new). Reminding yourself of this will put you in a position for increased empathy and cue you into a compassionate reality check that you and your client are connecting on a similar experience in real time. Finally, remember your breath is your best friend. Mindfully slow down your breathing and take deep belly breaths to center yourself and reset your physical and mental states. These guidelines will support you in getting out of your own way and putting your focus and attention more fully on your client.

ENGAGING IN 4-2-6 BREATHWORK

There are many variations of relaxation exercises and breathwork, so you are encouraged to research different methods and experiment (e.g., alternate nostril breathing, progressive muscle relaxation, guided imagery, etc.). These exercises are good to regularly practice on your own, as are helpful wellness strategies to share with your clients. The following basic and brief 4-2-6 breathing exercise can be used to help you center yourself and invite relaxation. This can be used to center yourself before and after a session, and discreetly during a session should you feel the need. The more you practice this exercise your body will begin to develop an efficient response time for relaxation, where one cycle of this breath can induce deep relaxation (think of this as classical conditioning to your advantage!).

Begin by placing both feet flat on the floor, and gently engaging your core so that your back is supported and your spine is long. Your hands can rest on your lap, palms down. On an inhale, slow-

ly roll your shoulders up, back, and on an exhale lower them down, noticing the space this creates in your center body. Tuck your chin slightly so that your spine is neutral. You can place one hand on your belly as you take a deep breath in through your nose, filling your lungs as your belly expands. On a slow exhale, feel your navel press inward toward your spine. Set your breaths to a count of 4-2-6. Inhale deeply counting to 4. Notice the breath rise from deep within your belly, to your lower ribcage, chest, throat, perhaps even through the top of your head. At the top of the breath, hold for a count of 2. Slowly exhale to a count of 6, mindfully riding the breath down from top to bottom. You may even notice that your exhales create a vibration in the back of your throat that resemble the sound of soothing ocean wave. Repeat this 4-2-6 breathwork a minimum of four times.

*See Personal Activity Exercise at end of chapter to support continued practice with another person in a virtual setting.

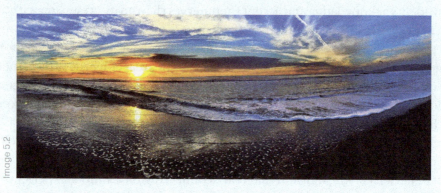

Image 5.2

Imposter Syndrome

The term *imposter syndrome* has been defined as "the persistent inability to believe that one's success is deserved or has been legitimately achieved as a result of one's own efforts or skills" (Lexico, n.d.). It is a common experience, in that an estimated 70% of adults are likely to feel this at some point in their lives (Sakulku & Alexander, 2011). As a counselor-in-training, if this situation is at play, you may have thoughts such as these:

- "I do not know enough to help this person."
- "I am not yet ready/competent to be a counselor."
- "We are so different in (age/culture/racial background/gender identity/sexual orientation/life circumstances/etc.) they will never accept me as their counselor."

The list could go on, but you get the idea! When thoughts like this creep up, it takes the focus away from your client and your relationship with them. In a nutshell, you end up "in your own head" and missing out on the positive partnership with your client. Since it is usually the thoughts that will cue you that imposter syndrome is negatively impacting your process, let's consider how cognitive behavioral theory (CBT) can support us in working through this challenge.

Drawing from CBT, these thoughts are examples of the cognitive distortions of mind reading, or making assumptions. Remember, assumptions are not facts, so these thoughts are not facts. It is important in these moments to identify the thought, hit the pause button, and replace it with a healthy and productive thought that is based on facts. It can also help to use the CBT technique of asking yourself what is the worst thing that could happen if your thought was accurate. Perhaps the client would be resistant—but we have the skills to handle resistance! We can explore this with the client and open up a conversation about the process of counseling and how our skills will support the client in addressing their concerns and working on their goals. Or maybe they decide to prematurely terminate counseling; then we can either help them through that process or, if they simply do not return without contact, we can trust that they have learned something about who they prefer to work with and will find a better fit for them. This is a good time to remember that we can only control our own process and that people are always free to exercise their own free will.

With these strategies in mind, revisit the example of negative thoughts and consider alternate thoughts based on facts that can counteract them. What other potential thoughts and replacements would you add to this list?

Over-Reliance on Particular Skills

Over-reliance on particular skills is an area we often give feedback on when we are teaching skills courses with our students. Consider the following scenario, and imagine you are the client in this brief exchange:

COUNSELOR: What brings you in today?

CLIENT: I am extremely frustrated with my job. My boss ignores all of my efforts, and the only times I ever hear from him is either when he is piling on more work for me to do or he is criticizing me for the work I've already done. I get excellent feedback from my customers, and it seems he doesn't notice or doesn't care.

COUNSELOR: How long have you been at your job?

CLIENT: 8 years.

COUNSELOR: Has the relationship with your boss always been this way?

CLIENT: Yes.

As the client, how are you feeling right now? Do you feel a connection with your counselor? (Maybe.) Do you feel truly heard and understood? Validated? (We would think probably not). And this was only after three responses; imagine how as a client you would feel if this went on for the better half of the session! These are important questions to ask, so it is not the skill of questioning that is problematic, but rather the over-reliance on the skill. Now, the counselor in this scenario likely has all good intentions and is focused on gathering information. This is something we often see, especially when our students are role-playing conducting intakes and/or first sessions. We just can't miss the relationship piece! Balancing skills, such as providing reflections and paraphrasing, along with ensuring your nonverbals convey warmth and empathy will help you avoid over-relying on a particular skill and support building a strong relationship. Remember that clients will come back to counseling not because of the specific questions you ask but because they feel a positive connection with you that is built on trust, respect, and understanding.

Weak Collaboration

Oftentimes when the relationship appears to be strained or otherwise "off" we can trace the cause to a weak collaboration with clients. Think of collaboration as a sense of partnership in working toward a common goal. We can develop this sense of partnership both with our nonverbal and verbal exchanges with clients. For example, are we intentionally matching our clients closely in vocal tone, volume, and pace? Are our physical movements and posture well aligned? Are we using language that is similar in style? More directly (and we will discuss this in more depth later in the chapter when we cover problem identification and goal collaboration), are we working from the client's experience and worldview to understand the problem and potential solutions? If we find ourselves blazing full speed ahead and losing connection with our client, it is important to slow down and remember to put our client first. Tune in to their experience, their presence, their words, and get back on their page. If you catch yourself getting a bit too directive or moving too quickly, you may find your client starting to check out by looking away (why are they checking their watch for the fifth time in 5 minutes?), minimizing their responses, or giving a reason they need to leave early. They may not give you a confirmed next session, ending with a "I'll contact you to set something up." To avoid this from happening, always remember to put your client and your relationship with them first, walk in step with your client as opposed to thinking/being three steps ahead, and when mistakes happen own them fully and course correct.

In summary, get through these pitfalls to building and maintaining a healthy therapeutic relationship by remembering to breathe, engaging in positive self-talk, balancing your skills, and maintaining your focus on your client. When in doubt and you find yourself too wrapped up in your own head and out of synch with your client, remember this phrase and use it as your mantra whenever you need: Trust the process.

Trust the Process!

At its core, a strong therapeutic relationship reflects your professional support to help your client while adhering to and maintaining the integrity of the ethical standards of autonomy, nonmaleficence, beneficence, justice, fidelity, and veracity (American Counseling Association [ACA], 2014). Following are some high-level considerations that support a positive therapeutic relationship throughout the process:

- There is a trusting and confidential relationship where limits are adhered.
- There is a respect for clients, and professional boundaries are maintained.
- The purpose of the relationship is to focus on the client's presenting problems and concerns with minimal counselor self-disclosure.
- There is collaboration on a mutually decided direction for treatment.
- There is the use of therapeutic skills and theory that drives the practice.
- There is an agreed-on understanding of compensation for treatment.
- There is an agreed-on session schedule, time frame, and focus on boundaries of information only in the context of the session.
- There is a natural and agreed-on process of termination when goals are met.

Introducing the Case of Juan

Now that the importance of the therapeutic relationship is fresh in our awareness, let's turn our attention to applying relationship skills specifically in a telemental health setting. Review the case study provided. We will refer back to this for the remainder of the chapter.

This case study is based on a client that I (Rosanne) worked with via telemental health. All identifying information has been adjusted to protect confidentiality. Please use this case study throughout this chapter to assist with applying the skills to the specific client's story.

The Case of Juan

The following information was gathered from the initial client web form submitted when Juan requested a counseling appointment through the counselor's platform:

Juan is a 28-year-old male whose preferred pronouns are he/him and identifies as pansexual. He stated he shared his affectional identity to his family and friends many years ago and that they have been very supportive. He reports his mother currently is having some medical problems, and his father is healthy. There is a history of depression on the maternal side. Juan has been in a committed relationship with his partner for the last year and half. He has a master's degree and works in a corporate setting where he has excelled in his career. He reached out via telemental health due to having a difficult time managing the level of anxiety and depression in his life. Several days of experiencing anxiety and a depressed mood have been persistent over the last year, but no suicidal ideation is evident. The stressors in his life are connected with a potential career change, moving to a different area of the country, finances, and relationship maintenance with his family and partner. He has reached out for treatment via video, phone, and chat messaging through the counselor's online counseling platform.

After reviewing Juan's case, you might be asking yourself, "How will I establish a relationship with him via a telemental health environment?" If this is your first thought, you are thinking like a professional helper and have been taught the power of the counselor–client relationship. There is quite a lot of research that has emphasized the relationship establishment and maintenance within therapy as a primary factor that contributes to client success (Friedlander et al., 2018; Norcross & Lambert, 2018; Young, 2021). The therapeutic relationship is more important than theory or techniques used in counseling (Norcross & Lambert, 2018), and all theories emphasize the importance of the relationship no matter what theory is implemented (Duncan et al., 2010). This does not discount the importance of ensuring that you are learning and applying counseling theories and techniques, but if you do not establish a solid relationship, there is a likelihood for a client to not return to counseling after the first visit or to terminate early.

In the case of Juan, the therapeutic relationship begins even as the client is searching online for a provider. Clients may browse through a website, insurance company provider names, and/or your picture to examine positive facial features of support and examine biographical information about years of practice and specialty areas. The World Wide Web has made this process quite simple for clients to gather information on their provider, prior to even reaching out. Juan reported to me (Rosanne) that prior to choosing to reach out, he looked me up to see if I was a right fit, and then took the chance to complete the information form. Upon receiving the information form, I had to make a quick and educated decision regarding how to best respond to Juan's list of concerns to jump-start the therapeutic relationship. Every provider and company will have different ways for clients to reach out to you. This might be via an encrypted email, phone call through the computer or cellular/landline phone, webform, or via an information form.

You have learned (or will learn) about the essentials of foundational skills in your counseling skills class, and it is important that these skills resonate in the first contact with the client. First contact in telemental health is commonly in written format, unlike the traditional appointment setting via phone. As a result, how a counselor responds sets the tone for the therapeutic relationship. With the therapeutic relationship in mind, we must consider our promptness, listen and hear with clinical eyes to the text that is written, and consider our writing response tone (are we validating the client's experience while demonstrating empathy, warmth, and positive regard in a strictly professional manner?). Considering the brief information received from Juan, as noted in the case study, consider which of the following responses you would choose as an initial contact to get counseling started with Juan:

Option 1

Juan,

Thank you for reaching out to me. From your profile it sounds like you are struggling with anxiety and depression, but it does not sound like it is impacting your life too greatly. Wow, I am impressed that you have been with your partner for a year and half and doing so well. I do not often see clients that are in long-standing relationships and are so well educated. I am looking forward to working with you because I am sure we can have great conversations. I have time this week to work with you via chat, phone, or video. Please agree to the documents I send you, pick a time, and we can get started.

Warm thanks,

XXXX

Option 2

Good evening, Juan,

I am sorry it has been a few days for me to respond. As you can imagine, I am swamped with lots of clients, and this is not my only job, so I am juggling a lot right now. I read your profile, and although I have quite a booked schedule, I should have some 30 minutes to chat or have a phone session that I can squeeze in this week. Please agree to my informed consent and schedule and we can chat.

Thanks,

XXXX

Option 3

Juan,

Thank you for reaching out to me. I know it takes a lot of courage to reach out to a professional counselor to talk with when issues arise. From your questionnaire, it sounds as if you would bene-fit from a live chat, live video, or live text session. You indicated having some struggles with anxiety and depression that you reported being linked to stressors in your life. I think it will be important to talk through these in counseling. I have availability to work with you, and it is best that we select a specific calendar date and time to ensure confidentiality. I conduct 30- or 50-minute live sessions weekly via chat, phone, or video and check my messages at least twice a day.

Before proceeding with counseling, I require my clients to agree to the client information form that includes my informed consent document. Please complete those forms and submit them, and then we can correspond via message regarding a time that is good for your schedule this week.

Warm regards,

XXXX

I hope you read through each of them and really thought about how to respond to Juan. Now let's break down each option.

As you read option 1, there is a positive tone at the beginning with saying thanks for reaching out. There is a bit of empathy and validation regarding his experience of depression and anxiety. There was an attempt to affirm the relationship, but the tone shifts quickly to being personal and judgmental about the counselor's other clients by writing about his level of education and long-term relationship that seems vastly different than other clients the counselor has served. Then, there is a friendship tone set as the counselor expresses excitement about the conversations. The author goes back into business by saying to complete forms, pick a time, and get started. If you were Juan, would you feel this would be a professional or a personal relationship? Would you proceed to schedule an appointment for counseling? Why or why not?

Option 2 immediately sets a tone that the counselor is frazzled, overwhelmed, and nonresponsive. It is imperative that counselors get back to clients within 24 hours especially when working to establish the relationship with a client. The counselor makes the entire conversation about the counselor's personal stress and is not making the client's needs a priority. If you were Juan, would you want to get started in a relationship that seems rushed and inattentive to your needs? I don't think so!

Option 3 sets a professional tone in the beginning that carries through the end of the response. Empathy, warmth, and concern for the needs of the client are conveyed. Active listening and collaboration between client and counselor is demonstrated, and the client is aware of what is needed to proceed with an appointment. If you were Juan, would you feel a sense of connectedness and caring by this counselor? How quick would you be to respond back to this counselor?

Applying Counseling Skills in Telemental Health: Practical Considerations

If you chose option 3 from the prior exercise, great job! Juan has responded to your message, and you now have a live video session scheduled this week. It is a good time to refresh yourself on the counseling skills you have learned about in your training program. Table 5.1 covers common skills taught in beginning skills courses:

TABLE 5.1   Counseling Skills Refresher

Attending Skills	Exploration Skills	Advanced Skills
▪ Conveying empathy, acceptance, and unconditional positive regard ▪ Active listening ▪ Minimal encouragers ▪ Reflections ▪ Paraphrasing ▪ Summarizing	▪ Open questions ▪ Closed questions/ clarifications ▪ Probing ▪ Scaling ▪ Packaging	▪ Silence ▪ Countertransference/ transference ▪ Immediacy ▪ Self-disclosure ▪ Challenging

Again, this text is not focused on the teaching of these skills, so if you need to review the nuances of the skills please refer back to resources from your skills class or a solid online resource such as *20 Basic Counseling Skills to Become an Effective Therapist* (Sutton, 2021). If you are feeling overwhelmed at the thought of translating what you have learned into a virtual platform, rest assured there are more similarities than differences when it comes to applying skills across traditional and telemental health counseling formats. Across both formats, in addition to continuously attending to the therapeutic relationship (we warned you this wasn't going to be underestimated!), you want to also keep the three Cs in mind as you apply your skills:

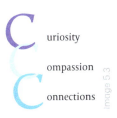

Image 5.3

- *Curiosity*—Maintain a posture of authentic curiosity as you aim to understand the client, their worldview, lived experiences, and goals for counseling.
- *Compassion*—Ensure that throughout your session, with each skill you use, that you are conveying compassionate responses to your client.
- *Connections*—There are many ways we can tune in for connections. For example, we can look to see the connections between aspects of the client's story (e.g., between past, present, and future experiences/goals), between aspects of self (e.g., strengths, challenges, beliefs, values), and between the client's wants versus needs.

With this in mind, let's return to the case of Juan.

Juan's appointment is Tuesday at 1:00 p.m. He was sent an automatic reminder of the appointment via the online management system the day before. The clinician sent a private message to the client the evening prior to the session reminding him to log on at least 5 minutes early to the session and to have a photo identification in hand for client verification. The clinician logs in 5 minutes before and sends a message to the client indicating she is online and will start the live video session as soon as the client is online. Once the client logs in, the clinician sends a message: "I am starting a live video session now, please accept." As Juan and the clinician connect, the counselor begins with a friendly greeting and verifies identity and online competence.

COUNSELOR: Hello, Juan. I am Rosanne. It is so great to see you here today.

JUAN: Good to meet you as well. I brought my identification for verification as requested in the appointment confirmation message you sent. I think this is a good idea since we are meeting online. I wondered how all of this worked.

COUNSELOR: Thanks so much for verifying your identity. It is so important that you and I start out this counselor–client relationship with this process so we can delve further into what brings you here. As you can see behind me, that is my licensure verification so we can both share identification with each other. I am wondering what you would like to know about my background before I tell you a bit about the counseling process.

JUAN: To be honest, I already looked you up online, so I read all about you, and it seems you have been a counselor for a while and teach people to become counselors as well? I feel like I picked the right person.

COUNSELOR: Well, great. I look forward to working with you. Before we get started, I want to verify that you are in a safe and confidential setting where we can talk without interruption and if you have any problems navigating this technology.

JUAN: Oh, yes, I made sure to schedule this when I am alone. Well, alone with my dog. I am very tech savvy, so this online format is ideal for me. I have good Wi-Fi and understand that if the internet goes out, we can shift to using the phone.

COUNSELOR: Great! Sounds like it is nice to have your dog with you while we work together. It is great to hear you feel comfortable with this technology. I do want to go over the informed consent process. I know I sent it to you so you could look over it and sign it. I will need to sign it as well after we review it together. What questions do you have from your review of informed consent?

JUAN: Yes, my dog, Brewster, rarely leaves my side! I am not sure what questions I have; once you go over it, maybe I will have more questions.

As we pull from this role-play, you can hear from this dialogue that there is a mix of relationship establishment along with completing ethical and legal requirements prior to shifting into completing the biopsychosocial/intake assessment. Let's do a quick checklist of what would be covered:

- Client identification
- Counselor identification

- Confidentiality in the clinical session
- Comfort with technology
- Informed consent

This dialogue ends with the counselor heading into the informed consent. Typically, the verbal back and forth of the components of the informed consent will take 5 or less minutes but can take longer with questions and securing signatures. After completing the informed consent, the counselor transitions into the biopsychosocial/intake assessment.

COUNSELOR: Now that we have completed the informed consent, I would like to get to know you a bit better and complete a thorough assessment so I can get a holistic perspective of your strengths and clinical needs. From your web form, it sounds like your partnership and work are things in your life that are really going well. You did indicate wanting to get assistance with anxiety and depression. Juan, I am interested in knowing a bit more about your struggles with anxiety and depression.

JUAN: I was not sure what to write on the web form, but I do think you captured what I was thinking at the time. I have been to counseling before, and it helped me, but the depression and anxiety continues to loom over me like a dark cloud.

COUNSELOR: I am glad I was able to capture what you expressed. I can picture how you describe depression and anxiety like a dark cloud over you and I am wondering how these storming emotions impact your life.

This begins the conversation back and forth between the counselor and client to make sure all the components of the biopsychosocial/intake assessment are complete. A great way to complete this online is to have one screen open with the client where you are visually connected and talking and another screen where the document is located and complete it as you collaborate with your client. I always let my clients know that I am writing and taking notes as we work together and that they have a right to review those notes. This is both ethical and legal. Once the biopsychosocial/intake assessment is complete, it is imperative to work with the clients to begin the process of the treatment plan by identifying problems and setting goals.

Identifying Problems and Setting Goals With Clients in a Telemental Health Setting

The moment you begin to take in the client's story, you are tuning in carefully to what the client needs from their perspective and where the change opportunities potentially lie. Identifying the problem is a key task that takes place early in your work with clients, and it is certainly a collaborative effort. As professional counselors, it is not our place to inform the client what the problem is. Rather, through a dialogue that encompasses the three Cs identified in the previous section, you will discover what is not working with the client and how the situation can be improved.

As you ask the various questions that emerge from the initial assessment, it is important to consider the interaction more like a partners' dance rather than as an instructor showing someone new how to dance. When partners are dancing, they stay within the rhythm and flow very naturally, working together and not against each other. With that type of process unfolding, the completion of the document will be more natural and flowing. Near the end of all of the elements of the biopsychosocial/intake assessment, it will be important to explore problems and identify goals. Look at how this might unfold between Juan and his counselor.

COUNSELOR: I appreciate you sharing so much about your life with me. I do hear that you had a history of anxiety since you were a teen and that your mother and father filed for bankruptcy. That can be quite a challenge for a teen to understand and cope with. As you progressed throughout college, your anxiety would emerge and impact you at varied times. You explored that you managed anxiety with exercise but there were times it did not work for you. You also reported that your mother took anxiety medication when you were a teen but that you were not as familiar with those details. Please let me know if I am on the right track.

JUAN: Yes, it is great to hear that you connected my anxiety to childhood events and how it impacts me now. That is so true in my life. I do not think I quite understand anxiety fully, but I know that with my anxiety I often get moments of feeling depressed as well.

COUNSELOR: I am glad I captured the connection to events and history of anxiety throughout your life. Anxiety and depression do go hand-in-hand sometimes, and when you have overwhelming anxiety, it can feel quite hopeless and also leave you feeling depressed. It seems as if you would like to focus on understanding this connection between depression and anxiety and feel improvement with both.

JUAN: Yes, I want to understand what depression and anxiety is, what happens in the body, and what will work to help me start feeling better. I hate feeling the way I have over the last 3 months. Another thing I need to work on is my people-pleasing behavior. I have such a hard time saying no to folks. These are all problems that have been impacting my daily life. Is it possible to have three goals that big?

COUNSELOR: Yes, we can definitely work through these three goals. Counseling is for you, and it is important to explore what you would like to focus on. I think that shows a great deal of insight into your needs. So, what I'm hearing you say is that your primary focus for counseling is maintenance of anxiety and depressive symptoms and implementing skills to set boundaries. Is this right?

JUAN: Yes, that is exactly what I want to focus on in our sessions. I am open to weekly sessions, if that is possible?

COUNSELOR: Yes, it is possible. We can go ahead and set some weekly times and begin the process.

Once the problem is clearly articulated, you will then work with your client to establish goals. Drawing from a common goal acronym used in CBT, you may consider using the SMART goals breakdown to map out clear and effective goals for counseling.

- **S: Specific**

  Write down the goal as specifically as possible. Let's say, for example, that Juan tells you that he just doesn't want to have such a high level of anxiety that he cannot function. You may be tempted to write "to not be anxious," but that is not a specific goal. Not being anxious could be a lot of things! Take a moment (put the book down so you can do this!) to consider alternatives. We'll wait.

  Let's say you narrowed down the field a bit by stating something like "to reduce anxiety." We will further clarify this as we keep following the checks in the rest of the acronym, but this is a good starting point. We can always adjust (with our client) as needed.

- **M: Measurable and meaningful**

  How will you measure whether Juan is achieving his goal? Is this tied to something he values and truly wants? What will a reduction in anxiety look like? After talking this through with Juan, he shares with you that his anxiety on a scale of 1 to 10 (with 10 being the highest) is at an 8 most days. Juan expressed that he felt that a level that he would like to get to is a 5. Discussing back and forth with a client about how an 8 manifests for him and what a 5 would look like is important. Using numbers in this way with a scaling question helps with measurability. In a video screen or in a chat format, the counselor can visually identify and list what Juan shares about what anxiety/anxiety management could look like at the different scale points. For example, Juan can offer a specific example for exactly what being at a 5 could look like versus a 1.

- **A: Attainable**

  Is Juan's goal attainable? How will he work toward this goal? What changes need to be made in order to meet the goal? If Juan identified a goal of zero anxiety, this is not attainable as humans are wired for anxiety to serve protective purposes. It is also not realistic to expect Juan to consistently reduce anxiety from an 8 to 5 in 1 week. It will take some time. We want to set goals that will have a successful outcome. So, Juan's attainable goal might be that he will report a reduction of anxiety symptoms from an 8 to a 5 in 3 months. Within that 3-month period, he will attain smaller goals along the way such as learning the cognitive, physiological, and psychological responses that exacerbate anxiety within a couple of weeks.

- **R: Realistic**

  Is this a realistic goal when we consider what Juan has shared with us about his experience? Looking over the information provided under specificity and attainability, we can see that it is realistic to think that Juan would report an anxiety decrease from 8 to a 5 in 3 months through the integration of specific interventions.

- **T: Time based**

  This is the Goldilocks factor in goal setting. If we aim too far off in the future, we run the risk of the client giving up on the goal or some other circumstance changing our plans before the goal plan comes to fruition. If we do not factor in enough time, we risk the client giving up due to frustration, feeling overwhelmed, or just not having enough time for the changes needed to take place. Either way, we must be careful to set the client up for success and not failure. We need to help our client find the "just right" time to plan for achieving the goal. Set a rational time-based goal as an initial benchmark to work toward, knowing that, together with your client, you can adjust as needed along the way.

As we explore the acronym SMART, focusing on one of Juan's goals (anxiety), we can lay out some long-term and short-term goals that are based on this method and lead toward the implementation of a theory. This collaboration on goal setting is done directly with the client (verbally with the client while in video or phone session or via chat function) and typed into the counseling record, which can be easily shared through an encrypted email and/or HIPAA-compliant online format.

Please utilize Table 5.2 to help draft a preliminary plan for Juan. The first one is completed as an example for you, with anxiety being the identified concern. After reviewing this example, consider depression and/or boundary setting as the identified concern and draft some possibilities.

TABLE 5.2 Preliminary Treatment Plan

Identified Concern	Long-Term Goals (e.g., 3, 6, or 9 Months)	Short-Term Goals	Theory or Intervention
Anxiety	Client reports a decrease in symptoms of anxiety from a 10 to a 5 within 3 to 6 months	1. Client will implement deep breathing exercises and progressive muscle relaxation in at least half of the incidences when anxiety is observed within the next month. 2. Client will implement cognitive reframing in at least half of the incidences when anxiety is observed within the next 2 months. 3. Client will report implementing preventive meditation measures and use of mindfulness 2-3 days a week over the next 3-6 months.	1. CBT 2. Mindfulness-based CBT 3. Psychoeducation of anxiety
Depression			
Boundary Setting			

The only way to gain proficiency at setting goals with a client is to practice the collaborative development of the goals with the client. Once these goals are established, the counselor and client will check in on progress each week. After the initial session documentation, the counselor will complete a weekly progress note indicating the client's progress, regression, or no change with goals. If goals are adjusted, this is documented as well.

Applying Counseling Interventions and Techniques in a Telemental Health Setting

At this point in your work with Juan you have established a healthy therapeutic relationship, collaboratively identified the target problem, and worked together to determine appropriate goals for counseling. We should say at this point that we also acknowledge that you have been and will continue to closely work with your clinical supervisor throughout the process. As you move toward intervention, review the following high-level checklist that applies across modalities and clinical presentations as you put together your case conceptualization/treatment plan, and then we will follow this with our application to Juan's case in a telemental health format.

Treatment Planning Checklist

- The selected interventions/techniques are theory based and informed by current literature.
- The selected interventions are sensitive to my client's cultural/ethnic background and unique needs.
- I am following ethical standards of competence by working within my scope of practice and training level.
- My clinical supervisor is closely monitoring my work, and I will reach out as soon as possible when questions/concerns arise.

Considerations for Intervention Delivery in Telemental Health

This is a good time to reiterate that there are more similarities than differences in the counseling process when comparing in-person and telemental health settings. We will take this opportunity to highlight some points specific to applying intervention within telemental health. We know, and have stated in prior chapters, that the most important factor in successful treatment is the quality of the therapeutic relationship. In telemental health, you have the opportunity to develop a strong rapport across multiple formats. Engaging with a client who is in the comfort of their own space, perhaps at more frequent intervals or during moments close to or during the time of the concern unfolding in real time (such as if using chat or email), can greatly facilitate the therapeutic bond with your clients. Another strength to the format is the ability to document key elements as you are engaging in counseling (e.g., secured email, transcript from a chat session, possible recording of video session [if this is in your practice and the client has authorized recording], and/or completion of assessments during the session). You can also leverage technology to implement interventions such as screen sharing to complete resources together (such as CBT worksheets), or engage in video-assisted exercises (e.g., mindfulness/relaxation work). As you work from a theory-based intervention, you want to ensure that your intentions and process are clear to your client. We find it helpful to prepare clients for what to expect before applying a specific technique or intervention. Let's look at how this could unfold with our hypothetical client, Juan:

> **COUNSELOR:** Juan, we've talked through how feelings of anxiety and depression are closely linked to our thoughts and behaviors. It can be very challenging to separate feelings from thoughts, especially when emotions are on the intense side. I have a worksheet that can help us practice doing this. Would you be interested in walking through it together?

> **JUAN:** Yes, that sounds interesting. Will you email that to me?

> **COUNSELOR:** Yes, I can email you the complete worksheet after the session. I'll also email you a blank copy so that you can practice more on your own in between sessions. For now, I'll pull it up in a screen share so we can complete it during this session.

The counselor shares a blank 4-factor worksheet and asks Juan to consider a recent event when anxiety or depression was high. The counselor guides Juan through each step, identifying the physical sensations, thoughts, feelings, and behaviors that were present during the event. As Juan explores his experiences across these factors, the counselor completes the worksheet, which is viewable to Juan, making sure to check with him frequently to ensure understanding and accuracy in what is being written. The counselor also takes the opportunity to dive deeper with Juan, such as exploring underlying beliefs that may be influencing his experiences. After the session, the completed and the blank forms are sent to Juan as promised.

VOICES FROM THE FIELD

What advice do you have for students who are considering a future practice in telemental health?

"My encouragement for students is to make sure to have a solid theoretical foundation first and then focusing on the attending skills by practicing them with people they are in contact with in their private lives. They can practice active listening and other attending skills in order to build the confidence to be able to use them online."

–Kelly James, PhD, LPC, NCC, Tulsa, OK

"The students have to realize that they possess the skills for telemental health in regards to connecting to the client and building rapport. I often hear the students say 'I do not have the nonverbal cues' and I always ask them what are the cues and how can they manifest differently so that you can understand what the client is needing. After doing internships through telemental health, I have them return to tell me that I was correct in that they did not miss the nonverbal cues."

–Alice Crawford, PhD, LCPC, Carpentersville, IL

"For students in online programs, do consider your experience as an online student. What do you like? What do you not like? What do you find to be the most effective form of communication? To a great extent, we are wordsmiths. With nonverbals becoming more limited and our energy not physically present in the space, we need to compensate somehow. Though we should never overdo anything to a point of being unnatural, do be intentional. Intentionally think through words, vocal tone, facial expressions, and how you conduct the session. This is as, if not even more, important than ever."

–Matt Glowiak, PhD, LCPC, CAADC, NCC, Bolingbrook, IL

Monitoring Therapeutic Progress Toward Termination

The therapeutic process is well underway, and you have a feeling that all is on track and moving along smoothly. Juan continues to return to counseling via weekly video sessions, and occasionally utilizes the chat feature briefly in between sessions. While a feeling is good, evidence is better! How will you directly monitor therapeutic progress? Three recommendations for tracking progress are to regularly elicit feedback from your clients, complete case notes after each session, as well as regular treatment progress notes, and administer intermittent assessment throughout treatment. Let's look at each of these methods in the context of Juan's case.

Regularly Eliciting Client Feedback

Client feedback is a natural part of each session with a client, and while eliciting feedback directly does not have to be in every session, it needs to be done periodically throughout treatment. It is important to always be preparing the client for termination. Here is an example of how to elicit feedback during a video session with Juan' after the fourth session:

COUNSELOR: Before we end for today, I wanted to take a few minutes to ask what your thoughts are about how treatment is going.

JUAN: I feel we are on the right track. I've been having less anxiety, and the use of mindfulness and tracking thoughts has really been helpful. I would like to continue monitoring how I am doing with anxiety but begin focusing more on depression and boundaries.

COUNSELOR: So, I'm hearing you say that the sessions have been useful and you've experienced progress with your anxiety by the use of mindfulness and tracking thinking. That is great to hear, and I can see that you are proud of your progress! In our next session, we will transition more into the depression symptoms you are experiencing lately, and your goal of setting boundaries.

Session Case Notes and Treatment Progress Notes

As you are aware from your skills and theory classes (or will be!), there are different ways to track progress. Each agency will have their own method of tracking progress. We will show the SOAP note format with an example from a session with our hypothetical client, Juan. Please keep in mind that wherever you complete your practicum and internship, there will be varied ways to track progress. Forms such as the one provided can be a digital version within the telemental health program used, or you can opt to type it up weekly in a Word document and save to the client's file.

SOAP notes are generally completed during or at the end of a session with a client. Due to the ethical importance of documentation (ACA, 2014), it is encouraged that the SOAP note is completed while in the session with the client or before seeing the next client.

Client name: Juan
Date of service: 1/3/22

Session starts: 4:30 p.m.   Session Ends: 5:20 p.m.

Type of counseling:

Individual _____   Couple _____   Family _____   Group counseling _____

Format:

In person _____   Video session _____   Phone _____   Chat _____   Email _____

S = Subjective complaint: Presenting problem(s) or issue(s) from the *client's* point of view. What the client says about causes, duration, and seriousness of issue(s). If the client has more than one concern, rank them based on the client's perception of their importance. It is a good idea to quote the client.

Example: "I've had a great week. I can feel my anxiety becoming more manageable."

O = Objective finding: Counselor's observation of the client's behavior during the session. Verbal and nonverbal, including eye contact, voice tone and volume, body posture. Especially note any changes and when they occur (e.g., a client who becomes restless in discussing a topic or whose face turns red under certain circumstances). Note discrepancies in behavior.

Example: Client presented with a good affect and mood. He has been practicing mindfulness and thought-tracking skills. He demonstrated insight into the link to his anxiety response and was open to receptive to CBT work.

A = Assessment of progress: Counselor's assessment of progress since last session and during the current session. Continual evaluation of client in terms of emotions, cognitions, and behavior. Include your hypotheses, interpretations, and conceptualization of client. Some counselors note the interventions applied in session and how the client responded to it.

Example: Juan is calm, focused, and enthusiastic about treatment. He demonstrated progress with anxiety from an 8 to a 6, his cognitions regarding events, and worked in session to review thought tracking over the week and to focus on the skill of cognitive restructuring in session.

P = Plans for next session: Plans for *client*, not for the counselor. Short- and long-term goals. How you want to interact with client; what you may plan to respond to in next session with client (follow-up on family issues discussed). Do you plan to help client focus on thoughts, feelings, or behaviors? What particular strategy or theoretical approach might you use? What do you base your plan on?

Example: Client will return to counseling in 1 week and bring back the though- tracking notes and report on cognitive restructuring and mindfulness use.

It is imperative to review the SOAP with the client before the next session so progress and treatment plan are assessed and the counselor can pick up from the last session.

Use of Assessments

With evidence-based treatment, tracking client progress at different intervals in the process is a systematic way to evaluate whether the treatment protocol is effective toward achieving goals. You can utilize both formal assessments (e.g., structured/manualized/standardized), as well as informal assessments (e.g., scaling, open questions). Using assessments intermittently through treatment is helpful in determining the "A" (assessment) of the SOAP note. For example, in Juan's case this may include an anxiety assessment prior to beginning session 2 (serving as the pretreatment assessment) and then tracking it again in 1 month (serving as the midpoint assessment) and then finally or shortly after at termination of counseling (post-treatment assessment). Following are two examples of how the counselor may introduce the use of assessments with Juan. With the first example, this shows how the counselor, during a live video session, could introduce the assessment plan. With the second example, the counselor engages with the client in a delayed messaging system (e.g., email or chat).

Example 1: During a Live Video Session

COUNSELOR: Juan, one thing I like to do throughout counseling is to use assessments to track your progress. So, before we begin our formal session today, since we completed the intake last session, I would like to get you to answer a quick self-report assessment regarding your anxiety. Then, we will use this same assessment to track your progress midway through treatment and at the end of treatment prior to termination. What questions do you have for me about this assessment?

JUAN: I like this idea because it can help me see my progress in counseling. If I could look at it, then I might have some questions about how it works.

COUNSELOR: No problem! I will send this to you right now in a private message using the online platform. You will see directions with the assessment. Please let me know if you have any questions as you review it.

Example 2: During a Delayed Message Interaction

COUNSELOR: Good morning. It was a pleasure to get to know you during our intake session. I know it was a lot of information, but I feel we now have a good plan of action to proceed. We discussed your goal of managing anxiety, and it is important to track your progress as we work together. Attached is a self-report anxiety assessment. I would like for you to complete this assessment and get it back to me prior to our next session. We will use this same assessment to track your progress midway through treatment and again prior to termination of counseling. Please review it and let me know if you have any questions.

JUAN: Sorry I am just getting back to you. It has been a hectic week at work (you'll hear about it in our next session!). Looking at the assessment, it is quite self-explanatory. I will complete it prior to our next session and get it messaged to you for your review. I think this is a good idea to see how I have progressed.

Monitoring client progress is a critical part of treatment. It is an ethical and legal requirement to maintain up-to-date records. As a future counselor, you need to consider how you would track weekly progress using appropriate record keeping along with documentation of an assessment as a tracking method. When applying these skills in a telemental health setting, navigation of the assessment and notes is at your fingertips, but it will be critical to consider your typing skills, options for use in a double-screen system, and always having documents ready. You can easily have self-made assessments ready along with blank DAP or SOAP notes that can be easily saved on a secure drive and completed during sessions. See Chapter 6 for more information on documentation on client progress.

Referral/Termination

There are times within counseling when a referral is needed. This might be for couple's counseling, a benefits program, or a medical doctor. In these situations, it is imperative to have a release of information on hand for you and the client to sign electronically.

Once that is completed, you might do a verbal call to the referral or provide an electronic letter via encrypted email. It is important that when a letter is completed your client reviews it prior to it being sent to an agency or third party. This fosters transparency and trust, as well as minimizes the potential for errors. Counseling begins with termination in mind. The goal of counseling is to help clients grow, and with that growth the client will be able to apply the new knowledge in everyday life without a need for ongoing counseling. Having termination in mind goes back to our previous section on tracking progress. Monitoring progress using verbal feedback, documentation, and assessments sets a precedent for the importance of progress and treatment termination.

Chapter Summary

In this chapter, we emphasized the importance of having a strong therapeutic relationship as the foundation for delivering clinical skills in a telemental health setting. It is common for counselors-in-training to feel uncomfortable as they begin working with clients, and this feeling can be heightened when doing so in a virtual setting. There may be concerns about the technology itself, your ability to connect interpersonally and authentically with your client, and/or concerns about your client's connection with you. The good news is that with proactive planning and a reliance on the counseling skills you have been trained in these concerns are likely to alleviate as you gain more experience.

No one starts out any skill at an expert level, so as you develop your expertise in counseling, remember to give yourself grace and compassion as you learn from each experience you have. Leverage the technology you have now (e.g., video platforms, chat) to communicate mindfully and demonstrate your counseling skills as you practice with peers and others in your life. As you go through each class in the program curriculum, we recommend that you find a study buddy to partner up with and schedule time virtually to connect and practice with one another what you are learning. Even better, pull together a small group of three or four so you have the added benefit of role-playing the counselor and the client and having one to two other peers to offer objective feedback as observers. You are investing in your future, so make the most of your training by seeking out every opportunity to put into practice what you are learning. We encourage you to have a plan to make the most of your time together as you practice with your peers. You now know that telemental health encompasses different modalities such as video, chat, phone, and email. For your practice time while you are learning skills, we recommend that you focus on using video sessions with your peers. This will give you the benefit of attending to the visual cues from your study buddy (referred to from this point as the role-play client [RPC]).

Ask your RPC to think of a scenario to role-play that is appropriate for the exercise. You aren't doing actual counseling, so we wouldn't want to enter the territory of crisis or highly triggering issues. Common examples students often use are general relationship concerns, role strain, mild/moderate anxiety, and so forth. Walk through the process with your RPC of highlighting the informed consent (assumed the RPC read it beforehand) and going over the limits to confidentiality as they are specific to your state's requirements. Then practice delivering your skills to develop rapport, understand the RPC's concerns, collaborate on goals, and work from a theory-based strategy to practice intervention techniques. These practice sessions can highlight some or all of these things in a given session, and it is important to focus your practice on the specific skills you are covering in your classes. Reflect on how doing these exercises is similar and different between virtual platform and in-person settings, and how you are developing your confidence to be competent in both modalities. If you find yourself getting stuck along the way, reach out to a trusted faculty member in your program or your clinical supervisor (if in fieldwork) for support. They are there to support your development as a professional counselor, and that includes preparing you to practice in a digital world.

PERSONAL REFLECTION ACTIVITY

Earlier in the chapter, you practiced engaging in mindful breathwork (4-2-6 breathing) to invite relaxation. You are now encouraged to extend your practice by sharing this beneficial exercise with another person! A script is provided for you to work from or adapt as you see fit. Since our goal in this book is to support you as you build your virtual helping presence skill set, you are asked to engage in this activity within a video platform (e.g., Zoom, Skype, Microsoft Teams, etc.). Start with a trusted person like a close family member or friend to gain comfort in walking another person through the activity. This would also be a great exercise to do with your RPC in your practice sessions! Remember, this isn't conducting therapy, so it is important to be clear that you are looking for volunteers to support you as you work on your skill of facilitating a relaxation exercise with another person. You could also benefit from asking a faculty member or supervisor to observe you as you do this skill for feedback. One option is to record yourself and send them your video to review. Make sure they know you are looking for candid feedback so that you can improve your work on supporting others in their wellness. When you finish the activity, respond to the following self-reflection questions:

- Did you experience any challenges in facilitating this exercise in an online setting?
- What went well for you that you want to maintain (e.g., vocal tone, setting up a session with a partner, technology considerations, etc.)?
- What will you adjust to improve the process?

Script For Guided Relaxation Exercise

Begin by placing both feet flat on the floor and gently engaging your core so that your back is supported and your spine is long. Your hands can rest on your lap, palms down. On an inhale, slowly roll your shoulders up, back, and on an exhale lower them down, noticing the space this creates in your center body. Tuck your chin slightly so that your spine is neutral. You can place one hand on your belly as you take a deep breath in through your nose, filling your lungs as your belly expands. On a slow exhale, feel your navel press inward toward your spine. Set your breaths to count of 4-2-6. Inhale deeply counting to four. Notice the breath rise from deep within your belly to your lower ribcage, chest, throat, perhaps even through the top of your head. At the top of the breath, hold for a count of two. Slowly exhale to a count of six, mindfully riding the breath down from top to bottom. You may even notice that your exhales create a vibration in the back of your throat that resemble the sound of soothing ocean wave. Repeat this 4-2-6 breathwork a minimum of four times.

*When complete, check in with your partner to see how they are feeling as a result of the exercise. Process any before/after shifts they may have experienced. Encourage them to practice at least once a day and to notice if they experience a difference in overall mood.

References

American Counseling Association. (2014). *2014 ACA code of ethics.* Author.

Duncan, B. L., Miller, S. D., Wampold, B. E., & Hubble, M. A. (Eds.) (2010). *The heart and soul of change: Delivering what works in therapy* (2nd ed.). American Psychological Association.

Friedlander, M. L., Escudero, V., Welmers-van de Poll, & Herrington, L. (2018). Meta-analysis of the alliance-outcome relation in couple and family therapy. *Psychotherapy, 55,* 356–371.

Hilty, D. M., Maheu, M. M., Drude, K. P., Hertlein, K. M., Wall, K., Long, R. P., & Luoma, T. L. (2017). Telebehavioral health, Telemental health, e-therapy and e-health competencies: The need for an interprofessional framework. *Journal of Technology in Behavioral Science, 2,* 171–189.

Lexico. (n.d.). *Imposter syndrome.* https://www.lexico.com/definition/impostor_syndrome

Norcross, J. C., & Lambert, M. J. (2018). Psychotherapy relationships that work III. *Psychotherapy, 55,* 303–315.

Sakulku, J., & Alexander, J. (2011). The impostor phenomenon. *International Journal of Behavioral Science, 6*(1), 75–97.

Sutton, J. (2021). *20 basic counseling skills to become an effective therapist.* Positive Psychology. https://positivepsychology.com/counseling-skills/

Young, M. (2021). *Learning the art of helping: Building blocks and techniques* (7th ed.). Merrill Counseling Series.

Credits

IMG 5.1: Source: https://pixabay.com/illustrations/internet-laptop-computer-notebook-1028794/.

IMG 5.2: Source: https://pixabay.com/photos/beach-sunset-panorama-panoramic-1846040/.

CHAPTER 6

Documentation and Billing in Telemental Health

Lisa Giovannelli

If it is not written down, it does not exist.

–Philippe Kruchten

Learning Objectives

After reading this chapter, you should be able to do the following:

1. Describe documentation needs specific to the practice of telemental health counseling
2. Identify ethical standards relevant to record keeping and communication practices in telemental health counseling
3. Discuss record maintenance and electronic billing practices in telemental health practice

Introduction

Telemental health counseling is on the rise, and therefore it is essential for counselors to increase their knowledge about the nuances of distance counseling and understand when and how telemental health services should be utilized (National Institute of Mental Health [NIMH], n.d.). Telemental health can aid

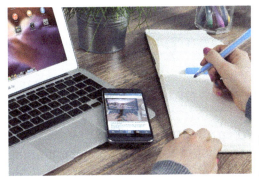

Image 6.1

133

in removing barriers, especially for those individuals residing in rural communities or for underserved populations with limited access to mental health services, and can help reduce the stigma for other populations, providing an added layer of privacy by attending counseling in the comfort of their own homes (Luxton et al., 2016).

The goal of this chapter is to increase counselors-in-training' knowledge about documentation and billing practices for telemental health. We will explore the various types of records that should be maintained for each client, including client profile, informed consent, releases of information, case conceptualizations, progress notes, assessment results, and assessment and documentation of safety issues. This chapter will also address some of the ethical considerations that coincide with documentation and maintaining records. More specifically, this chapter will focus on the ethical and legal issues related to communications and correspondence with clients or other professionals and record maintenance by providing basic knowledge of how to go about addressing these issues. One final goal for this chapter is to discuss some of the necessary steps counselors need to take to file insurance claims and to increase your knowledge about electronic billing practices.

Although I now have been a practicing mental health counselor for over 20 years, I recall when I first started learning in the field and significantly lacked skills in documentation. I recall the abundance of feedback I received from instructors and supervisors on how to work toward developing more refined and professional documentation. At times I thought it would never end, but alas, all that hard work paid off! I am now in the position of teaching students to work toward developing skills when documenting and writing case conceptualizations and case notes. While I have developed my own skills, I want to emphasize the importance of always being open to learning. It is good practice to continually ask yourself, "Can we ever really learn enough?"

I remember when I first started my private practice. I finally developed skills to write more professionally, and yet I felt I knew absolutely nothing about billing practices. Clearly, I still had a lot to learn! I continued to research and watch videos on best practices when filing claims and billing. One website I found very helpful was the American Counseling Association's (ACA) website. One of the members kindly posted a multitude of videos that walked the viewer through each stage of the billing process; it was amazing! I hope to guide you through some of the best practices for documenting and billing when performing telemental health, while encouraging you to always seek opportunities for continued learning!

Types of Records

When using telemental health as a means of providing counseling to clients, the counselor should ensure they are maintaining an adequate amount of information about the client. Some of the types of records should include a client profile (can be referred to by other names such as client information sheet), informed consent, releases of information, progress notes, assessment results, assessment and documentation of safety issues and case conceptualization. The following provides a more in-depth look at each type of record.

Client Profile and Initial Intake

During an initial contact with the client, we first want to develop the client's profile, which will include documentation of the client's demographics and initial intake information and determine whether they are appropriate for telemental health services. Before completing the client's profile, it will be important to take the time to assess the client's abilities and determine whether they are able to utilize the necessary technology to benefit from distance counseling, have impaired judgment, or pose as high risk (Ramirez et al., 2020). If a client presents with limited cognitive capacity or lacks appropriate technology skills, one option could be to include a care provider or guardian who can help facilitate the session for the client. In this instance, it would be necessary to address this in the informed consent as well as to obtain a release of information for the client's care provider (which will be discussed more in depth later in this chapter). If a client is deemed not appropriate for telemental health counseling, we can suggest the option of seeing them face-to-face or make any other necessary referrals for the client so that they can best meet their mental health needs in a more appropriate and comfortable setting.

The first record in counseling is generally the client's profile or initial intake information, which is typically completed prior to the initial diagnostic session with the client. During initial contact with a client or referral source, you should obtain basic information about the potential client. The client's profile will include information such as the client's address, telephone number, birth date, social security number, email address, and form of payment. When obtaining the telephone number, you will also want to ask whether you are able to leave voice or text messages on that number. Gaining permission to leave messages allows the counselor to contact the client via voice and text message when confirming appointments or for various other correspondence. Regardless of gaining this permission, counselors should make an effort to maintain the confidentiality of the client when leaving voice or text messages. For example, to protect client confidentiality, the counselor can leave a message that simply reminds the client about the appointment day and time but no other information that could identify the type of services being provided. For example, you could say, "Hello Joe; this is a reminder that you have an appointment scheduled for Monday January 1, 2020, at 12:00 p.m." Notice in the example neither the name of the facility nor the counselor's identity is provided. This helps maintain the client's confidentiality in the event someone else receives the voicemail or text message. Regardless of whether a client gives permission to leave messages (written or verbal), always make every effort to protect the client's confidentiality and be sure to document the fact that you have gained permission to leave such messages. Keep in mind that every facility will have their own policy for leaving messages with clients, so it is important that you acknowledge and follow their policy.

If the client is a minor, you want to ensure that you gather pertinent information about the parent or guardian, including essential contact information and relationship to the client. If the minor client resides with only one parent or there is indication of sole custody, be sure that you follow all legal and ethical practices, which could include having to secure a copy of the custody agreement to know which parent or guardian is permitted to consent to the minor's treatment (CPH & Associates, 2007). This is possible in a telemental health setting by obtaining the contact information of parents and/or guardians and emailing, calling, or conducting a video session to verify the pertinent documents. Further, know your state's laws regarding minors seeking treatment without parental consent. *Have you ever wondered whether minors are allowed to seek counseling services without parental consent?* In many states there are laws regarding minors being able to seek mental health counseling services without parental consent; however, these laws vary from state to state with regard to the age of the minor, length of services, and information pertaining to high-risk or medical issues. More information on working with minors in telemental health is provided in Chapter 7.

During this initial contact with the client, it is important to work toward confirming the identity and location of the client and providing the client with your license information (and your clinical supervisor's credentials while in training) so that they can verify your identity as well. Regarding initial contact, the first session ideally takes place face-to-face in the telehealth platform to verify the client's identity (i.e., being on screen visually). The National Board for Certified Counselors (NBCC, 2016) and the Association of Marital and Family Therapy Regulatory Board (AMFTRB, 2020) suggest that, whenever possible, the counselor should take reasonable steps to confirm the identity of the client, their location, and the client's preparedness for each session. Confirmation of the client's identity occurs by obtaining a copy of a photo ID and confirming that all information is up to date, including any name changes (e.g., changes due to marital status) and the address. All of this can be achieved during the initial contact with the client when developing the client's profile. In fact, it is recommended that client identity and their current location be obtained at the beginning of each session to ensure the client's location has not changed and no one is attempting to impersonate the client (Ramirez et al., 2020).

Assessing the client's preparedness for each session is essential to ensure the client is alone in a secure place, but also to ensure their confidentiality and safety. Further, by confirming their current location, should this be different from their home address that was previously confirmed, ensures the client's safety and allows you adequate time to search for local crisis numbers while in session in the event the client becomes high risk and requires crisis intervention (Ramirez et al., 2020).

The American Counseling Association (ACA, 2014) encourages counselors to confirm the identity of the client using a verification system, which can be agreed on during the initial meeting and can include the use of code words, numbers, or nondescript identifiers. For example, you can establish a verification system that would require your client to confirm their identity by stating their date of birth or the last four digits of their social security number. A code word can also be established to confirm identity across different digital platforms (e.g., handheld media device).

As a counselor-in-training (i.e., pre-licensed professional), you will need to let your client know who is supervising you and their licensure and background information. Your clients need to be informed that your clinical supervisor will be the licensed counselor overseeing their case. Therefore, it is imperative and ethical to inform your client that you are a counselor-in-training and always take steps to not misrepresent yourself as a licensed counselor.

Counselors must be aware of the laws pertaining to the states in which they are licensed to practice telemental health (ACA, 2014; AMFTRB, 2020; HPSO, 2021; Luxton et al., 2016). For example, I am licensed in both Ohio and South Carolina, which means I am currently only able to provide telemental health services to residents in Ohio or South Carolina based on the law and rules in both states. You should also be knowledgeable about the educational requirements and specific training that might be necessary in each state and not assume that all state requirements are the same (AMFTRB, 2020; NBCC, 2016). As a student, if you are seeking to include telemental health services as part of your training experience, first review your state requirements. Then make sure your specific program will allow for this experience. If so, make sure your intended clinical supervisor is very clear on state requirements for telemental health practice (and obviously, experienced!).

Informed Consent

It is always required to obtain the client's consent prior to providing any form of counseling, including telemental health counseling (HPSO, 2021). The informed consent is one of the most important documents the counselor will need when providing counseling since this is the client's consent to treatment. Obtaining consent for mental health treatment is a necessary and ethical standard of practice prior to initiating care (ACA, 2014; Luxton et al., 2016). It is important to acknowledge the differences between a typical informed consent and one that addresses issues unique to providing distance counseling (HPSO, 2021). As recognized by ACA (2014), a typical informed consent should include but is not limited to the purpose of counseling; goals; explaining the risks and benefits of interventions and procedures; counselor-in-training and supervisor qualifications, including relevant experience and credentials; counselor-in-training approach to counseling (e.g. theoretical orientation); continuation of services should the client become incapacitated or pass away; and the role of technology. ACA (2014) identifies the following factors unique to distance counseling that should be acknowledged in the telemental health informed consent:

1. The counselor-in-training and their supervisor's credentials, practice location, and necessary contact information
2. The risks and benefits of distance counseling and use of technology in distance counseling
3. The anticipation of technology failure and information related to an alternative plan
4. Anticipated response time to correspondence
5. Discussion of crisis interventions in the event the counselor is not available
6. Acknowledged differences in time zone(s)
7. Discussion of how cultural or language barriers are addressed
8. The policy for when there is a denial by the client's insurance
9. Social media policy

Again, as a counselor-in-training, you need to outline the supervisor's information as well as your role while under supervision and to whom you must report client information. This informs the client that you will be sharing aspects of their personal information for the purpose of training and supervision, so they have the opportunity to give consent or not.

Release of Information

In any setting where counselors provide services to clients, confidentiality is of utmost importance (ACA, 2014). Counselors providing services via telemental health have the same mandate to report harm and protect vulnerable populations (Luxton et al., 2016). In the health care industry, releases of information can appear in many forms and for different reasons. The Health Insurance Portability and Accountability Act of 1996 (HIPAA) is a federal mandate that was designed to develop standards to protect sensitive client information from being disclosed and to protect the privacy and confidentiality of clients. The Centers for Disease Control and Prevention (CDC, 2018) identifies covered entities that are subject to the privacy rules, including health care providers, health insurance plans, health care clearinghouses, and business associates. The following sections will provide details about the type of information released for each entity.

Basic Release of Information

As previously discussed, maintaining the client's confidentiality is extremely important. As many counselors-in-training are aware, there are limitations to confidentiality that include a client considering harm to self or others, reported cases of abuse or neglect in vulnerable populations (e.g., minors, older adults, individuals with disabilities), or if the counselor is court ordered to disclose information about the client (ACA, 2014).

However, in the latter instance, counselors need to keep in mind their right to privileged communication. In the case of *Jaffee v. Redmond* (1996), the U.S. Supreme Court agreed on the decision that communications between counselors and their clients are considered privileged and therefore protected from forced disclosure (ACA, 2021; Remley et al., 1997).

A counselor can disclose sensitive information about the client if they obtain a release of information signed by the client (Berghuis & Jongsma, 2014). Keep in mind that agreeing to disclose certain information for the purpose of continuity of care or collaboration with other professionals or family members is voluntary and the client does not have to sign any releases of information. You should take the time to explain to the client the purpose for the release of information, any information that will be disclosed, that signing is voluntary, and that they can revoke the release of information at any time.

Health Insurance Plans

Counselors-in-training cannot bill for services since they are not licensed. When an intern works for an agency, the supervisor typically has a specific plan of action when working with interns and seeing clients. This might be a sliding-fee scale or clients who are seen pro bono or a specific rate for a client to work with an intern. Clients will likely present to counseling having insurance plans that cover part or all of their mental health needs. As a result, there needs to be information contained in the informed consent or a separate financial disclosure that the client agrees to and signs, giving permission for certain information to be disclosed to third-party payers or to work with an intern and not bill insurance. Whatever the client agrees to, the counseling supervisor and trainee should have a discussion with the client so that they are aware of their payment responsibility. One example that tends to arise regarding payment is if the client is concerned about the impact of a diagnosis. To explain further, some clients might be concerned about information being passed to their employer, family member, or active military who might be concerned that a diagnosis might impact their ability to continue active duty. If this is the case and the client does not agree to consent to third-party pay, be sure to document this in a miscellaneous note and provide any other pertinent information indicating how you informed that client and the client's final decision.

Health Care Clearinghouses

At some point in your future career as a licensed counselor, you might be responsible for submitting your own insurance claims. As such, some insurance companies do not allow claims to be submitted on their website, but instead request that you submit claims through a clearinghouse such as Navicure or Availity. This will be discussed later in this chapter when discussing billing practices. For now know that this information should be contained in the informed consent and that the client should sign to agree to release information to third-party payers; be aware that this can include filing claims through a clearinghouse and not directly to the insurance company.

Business Associate Agreements

When providing telemental health, counselors can utilize a variety of platforms. The choice of platform should be well researched, HIPAA compliant, and require a business associate agreement (U.S. Department of Health and Human Services [HHS], 2013). The business associate is an individual or entity that provides a service requiring disclosure or protection of certain protected health information (HHS, 2013). A business associate agreement is a contract that provides an added layer of protection against disclosure of client information and should contain adequate information related to the relationship between the provider and entity, indication that the entity will not disclose information beyond the terms of the contract, breaches of confidential information, and where and the length of time the recording will be stored (HHS, 2013). As a trainee, the agency where you intern in a telemental health capacity should ensure that the business associate agreement is in place.

Case Conceptualizations

Formulating a clinical case conceptualization is essential in counseling as it documents information related to the client's background, presenting concerns, focus area of treatment, treatment goals, and identification of interventions intended to meet the client's needs (Novoa-Gomez et al., 2020; Zubernis & Snyder, 2015). Counselors-in-training should be able to provide a very clear and concise case conceptualization of a client that directs treatment planning and can be discussed during supervision or consultation (Sperry et al., 2014). There are different ways to present a case conceptualization, so always abide by your training site's protocols. As one example, Sperry et al. (2014) suggests case conceptualizations include four components (diagnostic formulation, clinical formulations, cultural formulation, and treatment formulation).

Once the client has been assessed and you are working toward developing a diagnosis and treatment plan while being culturally sensitive, think in terms of extracting the most pertinent client information and work toward providing a clear and concise picture. Very simply, you want to take a lot of information and condense it. Another good rule of thumb is to remember that the most relevant information related to the client's presenting information and history should be cohesive in justifying a diagnostic impression that in turn informs evidence-based treatment and interventions.

EXAMPLE CASE CONCEPTUALIZATION COMPONENTS

1. *Diagnostic formulation* is a description of the client's presenting symptoms taking into consideration the nature and severity of these symptoms. Diagnostic formulation attempts to answer the question, "What happened"? This takes into consideration DSM-5 (APA, 2013) criteria (Sperry et al., 2014).

2. *Clinical formulation* is a longitudinal explanation of symptoms. For example, we want to answer how the symptoms developed, how the symptoms were maintained, and how the symptoms resulted in a dysfunctional lifestyle (Sperry et al., 2014).

3. *Cultural formulation* includes cultural considerations that contribute to the presenting concerns. Cultural formulations consider the client's cultural identity and level of acculturation and how these might impact the client's personality, development, and level of functioning (Sperry et al., 2014).

4. *Treatment formulation* collectively considers the diagnostic formulation, clinical formulation, and cultural formulation to determine what can be done to address these to work toward an increased level of functioning and a decrease in symptom presentation (Sperry et al., 2014).

When documenting a case conceptualization for telemental health, I have personally found it beneficial to utilize one of the more common practice software programs. These software programs often provide templates useful for documentation of client intakes, progress notes, and treatment plans. One thing to be aware of when using forms provided by different sources is that terminology may vary from what you have learned in the past. For example, some software programs use the term *psychotherapy intake note* rather than *case conceptualization* and have a template available to document all essential information contained in a case conceptualization. This particular diagnostic intake template requires documentation of the presenting problem, mental status, risk assessment, objective content, biopsychosocial assessment, cultural considerations, treatment plan, and diagnosis, which is similar to requirements for a case conceptualization. When providing a diagnosis, you may also be asked to provide a justification for the diagnosis (which is very good practice while you are in training!). If this information is documented in a clear and concise manner, as previously suggested, this document can then serve as means for communicating and corresponding with other health care providers. As a reminder, when sending any client information to other health care providers, you must obtain the client's written permission via a signed release of information.

Let's practice! Review the following brief case scenario and discuss each aspect of a case conceptualization, including the diagnostic formulation, clinical formulation, cultural formulation, and treatment formulation:

The client is a 41-year-old Hispanic female who presents with increased anxiety and depressive symptoms that reportedly started in March 2020 when the global pandemic took hold. The client acknowledged that her family relocated from Puerto Rico in 2018 and reported that while she experienced some difficulty with adjusting to a new culture, she resided near her family and only had to drive approximately 20 to 30 minutes to visit them. The client reported that since COVID-19 and the mandates to shelter in place, she could no longer visit her family due to concerns about the health and well-being of her aging parents. The client reported that she was used to seeing her parents and various family members on a regular basis, almost daily, enjoying their company during dinners and family gatherings.

The client acknowledged the following symptoms: increased sadness for most days, feeling hopeless, lack of motivation, frequent worrying, feeling tense and anxious, increased irritability, difficulty concentrating, and more recently panic attacks. The client stated that although some of the restrictions were lifted, she still fears contracting COVID-19 because not all people follow the guidelines for wearing masks. The client acknowledged that her symptoms initially presented after relocating from Puerto Rico; however, these were very mild. The client went on to report that her symptoms increased significantly upon hearing about COVID-19, more so during the lockdown, but have increased to an unmanageable level since some of the restrictions were lifted.

Connect with a small group of classmates to review the case and discuss the following:

- *Provisional diagnosis/diagnoses*
- *Clinical formulation*
- *Cultural formulation*
- *Treatment formulation*

Progress Notes (Case Notes)

Note that throughout this section the terms *case note* and *progress note* are used interchangeably. Some telemental health platforms might use one term or the other. Counselors-in-training must keep in mind that federal regulations pertaining to protected health information under HIPAA include securing client progress notes (Berghuis & Jongsma, 2014). Counselors are responsible for maintaining accurate and adequate documentation while at the same time ensuring maintenance of confidentiality (ACA, 2014; Wheeler & Bertram, 2019). The documentation of a client's progress note should occur as soon as possible following a session (Berghuis & Jongsma, 2014). However, it is highly encouraged to document any notes that address high-risk situations immediately following the incident (or as close as possible). For example, if a client presents with suicidal ideation, you and your supervisor will assess the level of risk and determine the most appropriate follow-up, including the development of a safety plan. This will be documented immediately following the session. The purpose for not delaying documentation of case notes related to high-risk cases is due to the fact that the individual and situation could potentially escalate. In the example, if the client leaves the telemental health session and ingests illicit substances or alcohol that results in compromised decision-making, they could follow through on suicidal thoughts that occurred during session. If this note is not documented and the client committed suicide after the session, your or your supervisor could be held liable. Always remember, if it is not documented it never happened.

Progress notes need to be written clearly and concisely. It can take time to develop these skills, so be patient with yourself and the process. Clinical note writing is intended for a small but often very professional audience, and therefore learning to write utilizing clinical and professional terminology is essential (Berghuis & Jongsma, 2014; Hodges, 2021). Given the importance of clinical case notes for the counselor-in-training, it is advantageous to your professional development to have a clinical supervisor review your notes until you become more familiar with what constitutes an appropriate case note.

DO'S AND DON'TS OF PROFESSIONAL DOCUMENTATION

The following example terms are typical mental status exam items that can be assessed during each session. Note the differences between professional and nonprofessional observations.

Terminology	Not Recommended	Recommended
Appearance	Client smelled bad and looked like they just got out of bed.	Client presented with poor hygiene; disheveled and lethargic
Behavior	Client looked like they were lying because they would not maintain eye contact	Client presented with avoidant eye contact; cultural values should be considered
Mood	Happy, very happy, sad, very sad, tired, angry, nervous	Euthymic, euphoric, dysthymic, dysphoric, lethargic, irritable, anxious
Affect	Client was initially very angry and obnoxious but later seemed happy and relaxed	Client presented with full affect, mood initially irritable, later presenting more euthymic and comfortable as evidenced by clinician observation that client became more open and willing to engage in session
Thought content	Client was hearing voices and seeing aliens, stating, "I am the ruler of aliens. I am their leader and I have superpowers."	Client presented with auditory and visual hallucinations and delusion of grandeur

While this is not an exhaustive list of mental status terms, this example is intended to assist you with learning ways to be more concise while utilizing professional terminology. To explain further, let us think in ethical terms when writing case notes and the possibility that your notes could be subpoenaed to court. Imagine that you are the counselor and you have a client that is going through a divorce and custody battle. Your client informs you that his spouse made allegations of domestic violence but assured you that the allegations are false. However, as you assess further you learn that the client and his college buddy were in a physical altercation during college while out at a bar one Saturday night. Your client goes on to inform you that he was merely defending his friend from aggressors. When documenting your case note, you include a notation indicating that the client informed you that he was in a "bar brawl" and state nothing further. If subpoenaed to court, could this note potentially cause harm to your client? In this instance, the spouse's attorney could suggest that the incident in college and current allegations of domestic violence indicate patterned behavior and therefore could result in potential harm to your client, despite the fact that he was merely defending a friend in one instance and that the allegations of domestic violence are merely due to his spouse's anger about the divorce and are reportedly false. After all, a rationale for privileged communication is that our clients trust our actions and that we will not disclose personal information that could be potentially damaging to them. While counselors are always aiming to "do no harm," we do need to keep in mind that we also have an ethical and legal obligation to maintain adequate and accurate records on each client (Wheeler & Bertram, 2019).

Assessments

Assessments are a routine and integral part of counseling. One of the first things counselors do prior to administration of any assessment tool is to consider their professional codes of ethics and determine whether they are qualified to administer a particular assessment tool. Assessments are integral for assessing the client's presenting problem, informing toward a diagnosis (but not intended "to diagnose"), supporting treatment planning, and evaluating client progress (Whiston, 2013). Counselors need to ensure they are qualified to administer a particular assessment (ACA, 2014; Balkin & Juhnke, 2018). One thing to remember is that most test publishers have qualification levels, including the following:

- Level A: Requires little to no formal training
- Level B: Might require a minimum of a master's degree and affiliation in a professional organization
- Level C: The highest level of qualification, which typically requires a doctoral degree in psychology or closely related field and specialized training (Balkin & Juhnke, 2018).

As a counselor-in-training, you may only be permitted to utilize those assessments recognized as level A. As a result, and so as not to practice unethically or beyond your professional scope of practice, always consult with your supervisors when considering administration of any assessment, whether you believe it is a level A assessment or not. When considering an assessment tool, counselors will need to first determine whether they are qualified, then ensure they choose one that is appropriate for the client by giving consideration to the presenting concerns and one that is culturally sensitive (ACA, 2014). Counselors also want to take into consideration the reliability and validity of any chosen assessment tool (Balkin & Juhnke, 2018). Ask yourself these questions:

- Is the assessment measuring what it is supposed to measure?
- Does the assessment consistently measure depression or anxiety and so forth?
- Is the assessment appropriate for a particular culture I am assessing?

Again, keep in mind that supervision and consultation are valuable and necessary when utilizing assessments in counseling, including during telemental health practice (Luxton et al., 2016). The choice of assessments, along with administering assessments as a counselor-in-training, should always be at the discretion of trainees' supervisors since having qualifications (e.g., beyond level A) while working toward licensure is not common.

Whether in person or via telemental health counseling, assessments can include the initial screening of the client, a biopsychosocial assessment, risk assessments, or utilization of various other assessments specific to the client's presenting symptoms. For example, if a client is presenting with depression, the counselor might want to consider an assessment tool that is reliable and valid for measuring depression. In telemental health counseling, assessment information can be collected by the client, family members, or other entities, either synchronously or asynchronously and using web-based assessment resources (and again, with client consent and authorization of release of information; Luxton et al., 2016). One issue to think about before getting started is to know that, unlike assessing a client in person, counselors have limited sensory interaction with clients during telemental health sessions (Ramirez et al., 2020). To discuss this further, think about how technology and distance counseling might limit our ability to hear, see, or smell. While this might not seem relevant, let us consider the mental status evaluation. Most often, the mental status evaluation will assess hygiene, appearance, and dress. But what if it is the case that the client has not showered for days due to experiencing depression? We cannot know this or assess this through all forms of distance counseling or use of olfactory sensory information. When assessing mental status related to gait and appearance, one suggestion is to have the client walk across a room in their home (Ramirez et al., 2020). While this might be a great idea, know that your visual might be impaired, and therefore your judgment and assessment of the client's mental status might not be as accurate. What is recommended is to document this information in your case note and inform your supervisor that there were limitations when assessing the client via the telemental health platform used.

If administering a web-based assessment, there should be thoughtful consideration to internet connection and variability in size or resolution of the web-based assessment tool, as some computers might produce smaller or larger images (Luxton et al., 2016). Be sure that you have a discussion with your supervisor and client prior to administration of web-based assessments. This discussion can consist of what to do in the event the internet connection is lost. You can also meet with the client prior to administration of a web-based screening to determine how this will appear on their screen and whether other options might be available if needed.

One other consideration for counselors is to have the client complete assessments on their mobile device using available apps. By using mobile applications, the counselor can obtain information regarding the level of the client's presenting symptoms that can be tracked and then analyzed remotely and in real time (Huxton et al., 2016). If utilizing this form of assessment, be sure to address this in the informed consent and identify any legal, ethical, or other issues that the client should be aware of beforehand so that they are fully informed and can consent. Be sure that you are aware of all federal or state laws regarding confidentiality and HIPAA requirements, as some state laws vary and an informed consent might not be adequate (Luxton et al., 2016). For example, HIPAA encourages risk assessments of technology, including mobile devices, which would require us to inform our clients of any risks to them should they utilize their mobile device; this could include issues related to confidentiality (Gilbertson, 2020).

One important consideration is whether the counselor should be present when a client is taking a web-based assessment or while completing an assessment on a mobile device. I believe that the counselor should be present during any administration of any assessment tool, which is consistent with ACA (2014) codes of ethics (E.7.d). ACA (2014) suggests that counselors appropriately use formal assessments relevant to the client's needs and that counselors should not administer unsupervised assessments except in rare instances. There are a number of reasons the counselor should be present during administration of all assessments, including being able to observe the client while they are being assessed. For example, imagine that you are at a clinical site and are asked to administer a depression assessment to one of your clients. As you are doing so, you notice that they seem to be struggling, and it appears as though they are taking a lot more time than is typical for this particular inventory. One very important question that should be asked prior to administering any questionnaire, assessment tool, or screening is to politely ask your client about and assess their reading level. In this instance, the client could likely be struggling because they cannot read the questions or do not understand the meaning. There are various possibilities why this could be a challenge for the client, including developmental level, cognitive abilities, culture differences, and so on. Another issue to keep in mind is how the client might respond to the results. Another important reason for being present while your client completes an assessment is for the purpose of monitoring any negative reactions and their safety. For example, imagine the client is presenting with depression, anxiety, or posttraumatic stress disorder and some of the questions trigger your client. Ask yourself, "Can I monitor important reactions if I am not in the session? Can I provide appropriate 'immediate' responses for my client if I am not present during completion of an assessment?" If we are present while our client takes the assessment, we can provide immediate and necessary interventions to ensure no harm to our clients and provide them with any follow-up instructions to further ensure their safety.

Counselors have the responsibility to discuss the results with the client (ACA, 2014; Luxton et al., 2016). If a client were to take an assessment without being supervised and interpret the results incorrectly or assume the worst-case scenario, this could result in harm to the client. Be sure you take the time to discuss this with your client for their own protection as well as your own. Each assessment tool will have its own set of instructions regarding how to administer it, the cost, and scoring procedures. With this knowledge, it is imperative that a supervisor has fully discussed with you the process of conducting assessments and discussing results with clients.

VOICES FROM THE FIELD

What has your experience been with adapting documentation for telemental health practice (e.g., clinical documents such as telemental health–specific informed consent/progress notes/authorization for release of information and billing documents/procedures)?

"I have always had the option of telehealth for long time clients so I already had paperwork to that effect. While it has been updated to reflect no more face to face, in person options, the updates were minor and able to be changed quickly. All informed consent is sent to the client before their initial session and it is understood that a password to attend a session will not be sent to the client until all paperwork is returned by a secure email to me first. Billing is taken care of up front through a scheduling site with a secure platform. Progress notes are all digital and secured on a computer in a locked office with password protections."

–Melissa Lee-Tammeus, PhD, LMHC, Jacksonville, FL

"Platforms offer ways for clients to access forms easily, and review in session with the opportunity to address questions. Notes are conducted in the same manner through the platform."

–Robin Switzer, LPC, NCC, St Louis MO

Assessment and Documentation of Safety Issues

While careful documentation of client records and information is essential, what is always of utmost importance is to consider the safety of your client. Further, while you might initially assess to determine whether a client is appropriate for telemental health, you have to continue to monitor if they are high risk because this might not become apparent until the client has already started counseling and later presents with safety issues, including suicidal ideation or intent. In addition, while we might perform a mental status evaluation during the initial diagnostic assessment, doing so again later could be warranted, and it may be good practice to perform this during each session (Luxton et al., 2017).

Ramirez et al. (2020) reported that COVID-19 in 2020 contributed to an increase in mental health–related issues as well as increases in domestic violence and suicide, identifying social isolation as a primary cause. Since it is suggested to assess mental status and suicidal risk during every telemental health session, one procedure for doing so is the use of the Collaborative Assessment and Management of Suicidality (CAMS), which is recognized to be useful in a variety of settings including telemental health (Suicide Prevention Resource Center, 2017).

TIME TO BOOKMARK!

Counseling students and professionals can access CAMS training to use with a variety of populations and in various settings: https://cams-care.com/.

Luxton et al. (2016) acknowledged that safety issues in telemental health are similar to those in an office setting but pose additional challenges, including behavioral emergencies (e.g., suicidal), medical emergencies, homicidal risk/firearms, or technical difficulties.

The process by which the counselor addresses safety concerns should be documented in the informed consent. This information can sometimes include a crisis intervention phone number and local crisis intervention facilities. However, the counselor should also keep in mind that emergency situations such as a pandemic can arise, and thus they should have a backup plan due to closures or other reasons when clients might not have access to necessary services at the time they are needed (Luxton et al., 2016; Ramirez et al., 2020). Luxton et al. (2016) propose the following categories as a guide for effective safety planning:

1. Assessing appropriateness for telemental health
2. Assessing client's risk factors
3. Plan for coordinating services with other health care providers
4. Developing a list of emergency numbers available for client
5. Assessing technology issues
6. A safety plan document with copies provided to the client and maintained in the client's records.

Record Maintenance

Counselors have an ethical and legal responsibility to maintain adequate record keeping, and failure to do so could result in malpractice and other legal actions (Wheeler & Bertram, 2019). Counselors must reasonably safeguard electronic protected health information (ePHI) from any anticipated threats to the security or integrity of protected health information (Chen & Benusa,

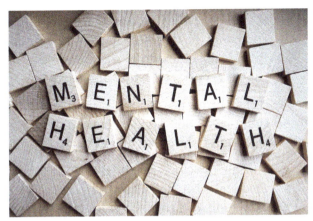

Image 6.2

2017; Lawley, 2012). Record maintenance includes assurance that client records are secure and protected from damage or loss and cannot be altered in any way (Wheeler & Bertram, 2019). Whether you choose to maintain records in a hard copy form or electronic format, these records should be legible, recorded in ink or electronically recorded, and contain the hand-written or electronic signature of the original author and a time stamp with the date the note was actually written (Wheeler & Bertram, 2019). Poorly maintained records can result in ethical violations and legal issues for any number of reasons (Lawley, 2012).

HIPAA has requirements for protecting hard-copy and electronic files. While it is suggested to maintain both physical and electronic files on all clients, if your supervisor chooses to maintain physical copies of client records, they should be protected by securing them in a locked file cabinet and adding an additional layer of protection by securing the locked file cabinets behind locked doors (ACA, 2014). Records should also be kept in an area where there is little chance for destruction to occur—for example, keeping the filing cabinets in an area where there is little to no chance for damage should a flood occur causing potential damage to the records, especially if hard-copy files are the only records you have. Not only are there suggestions or requirements to maintain physical copies of client records, there are additional steps that should be taken to secure records electronically.

The ACA (2014) code of ethics recommends that counselors take necessary steps to ensure the security of records through encryption. Therefore, it is necessary to seek guidance and educate yourself further to ensure ethical and legal compliance for securing client records. Counselors want to maintain electronic files with encryption as well as back them up for extra security (Lawley, 2012).The following information will provide some additional suggestions. Of course, consult with your supervisor first to ensure you are meeting legal, ethical, and agency requirements.

Chen and Benusa (2017) make the following suggestion for assessing integrity or risks to secure or transmit PHI:

1. Evaluate the likelihood and impact if a breach were to occur.
2. Following the risk assessment, take appropriate measures to secure data.
3. Provide documentation and rationale for security measures.
4. Update security measures and reassess as needed.

The Health Insurance Portability and Accountability Act (HIPAA) and the Health Information Technology for Economic and Clinical Health Act (HITECH), provide the following suggestions for securing records:

1. Storing on a cloud that is HIPAA compliant
2. Frequently backing up records, especially when new information is added
3. Use of software that allows limited access
4. Information encrypted at a location and prior to transmitting
5. Access that requires a two-step authentication process (Chen & Benusa, 2017; Lawley, 2012)

While counselors and other mental health and medical professionals might take all necessary steps toward securing PHI, there are unfortunate data breaches. Should a data breach occur, those entities securing the PHI must inform clients of the breach and about the possibility that their information has been compromised (Lawley, 2012). By law, if data was not protected and a breach occurred, a counselor is expected to notify clients within 60 days if the information was involved in the data breach (Lawley, 2012). While some of the larger facilities have individuals knowledgeable about technology and security requirements, many smaller practices do not. This can become an issue, especially if the professionals in the practice lack sufficient technology and awareness of PHI security laws, so it is highly encouraged if this is the case to hire a consulting firm and information technology specialist (Chen & Benusa, 2017).

Electronic Billing

While many counselors-in-training under supervision might not perform billing practices, the following will help provide a foundational understanding. As with record maintenance and electronic communications, electronic billing practices need to adhere to ethical and legal practices recognized by HIPAA regulations. There are several things a counselor-in-training must do before anyone is able to bill for those counseling services. One of the first things that I teach counseling interns is to apply for a National Provider Identifier (NPI). The NPI is a number you apply for once and use to identify you as the providing counselor when performing billing and submitting claims to insurance companies. I encourage you to ask your supervisor whether anyone at the facility has already applied for an NPI on your behalf (remember, you can only have one NPI). Once you have obtained an NPI, you can then submit your information to the nonprofit organization Council for Affordable Healthcare, Inc. (CAQH). CAQH is a database where providers submit professional information such as education, training, and professional experience. This is the website insurance companies will use to review your information to make credentialing determinations.

TIME TO BOOKMARK!

You can obtain an NPI at the following website: https://npiregistry.cms.hhs.gov/. You can apply for a CAQH identification number and submit your personal/professional information by proceeding to the following website: https://proview.caqh.org.

It is likely that soon after you complete all of your academic and clinical work in your counseling program (i.e., practicum and internship) your employer will want to begin the insurance credentialing process for you. Once you are credentialed with government-funded insurance such as Medicaid or private insurance companies, you or your employer can begin billing for client sessions and submitting claims to the insurance companies.

When submitting claims, this can be done a few ways. The typical billing form is the 1500 standard claim form, which is often used by medical and mental health providers. This form can be submitted electronically or in a physical hard copy via mail (although more often electronic billing is more efficient for all). Counselors can also utilize the insurance company's website to directly submit the form. Also, some insurance companies use clearinghouses. This means that claims are not submitted directly to the insurance company but are instead processed through the clearinghouses. Recall from the "Release of Information" section regarding clearinghouse and business associate agreements that this information needs to be discussed in the informed consent and that additional measures might need to be taken to maintain client confidentiality. Be sure to acknowledge the communication and correspondence requirements to ensure confidentiality and ensure legal and ethical practice.

As previously discussed, claims can be submitted online through a secure server on an insurance company's website or the clearinghouse's website. If a practice management is utilized, claims can be filed using this method. To enroll using a practice management system, you will need to complete enrollment forms for each insurance company, which then chooses a clearinghouse where the claims will ultimately be submitted. Counselors can opt to have remittance (reimbursements) sent via electronic funds transfer (EFT), but the counselor will also have to provide necessary banking information and forms for this to occur.

When filing claims for mental health services there are specific current procedural terminology (CPT) codes that we frequently utilize. The following CPT codes are recognized by most insurance when submitting claims for billing, and two of the most common include Diagnostic Evaluation (90791) and Therapy With Client for 60 Minutes (90837). You want to be familiar with other CPT codes, and when billing for telemental health you use the modifiers GT or 95. When billing for a telemental health session, the location type is documented as 02, which indicates distance counseling or medical services as opposed to 01," which is used as the location type for an office visit. While billing for mental health services can be tedious initially, once you grasp the concept, filing claims will progress with ease.

Chapter Summary

This chapter focused on increasing your knowledge about documentation and billing practices for telemental health. You learned about the various types of records that are maintained for each client, including client profile, informed consent, release of information, progress notes, assessment results, assessment and documentation of safety issues, case conceptualizations, and some of the related ethical considerations that coincide with documentation. This chapter worked toward providing some basic knowledge regarding ethical and legal issues related to communications and correspondence with clients or other professionals and record maintenance. As discussed throughout this chapter, always acknowledge additional ethical and legal considerations that might apply or change over time. This chapter also discussed some of the necessary steps you will need to take in order to file insurance claims and to increase your knowledge about electronic billing practices.

APPLICATION ACTIVITY

Imagine you are a counseling intern in a hypothetical group practice. Develop an informed consent for telemental health practice and present it to a faculty member in your program or your clinical supervisor for review and feedback.

References

American Counseling Association. (2014). *2014 ACA code of ethics*. https://www.counseling.org/resources/aca-code-of-ethics.pdf

American Counseling Association. (2021). *Confidentiality or privileged communication*. https://www.counseling.org/knowledge-center/licensure-requirements/confidentiality-or-privileged-communication

Association of Marital and Family Therapy Regulatory Boards. (2020). *Teletherapy guidelines.* https://amftrb.org/wp-content/uploads/2021/06/TS-Teletherapy-Guidelines-09.12.16.pdf

American Psychiatric Association. (2013). *Diagnostic and statistical manual.* (5th ed.). Author.

American Psychological Association. (2020, March). *Informed consent checklist for telepsychological services.* https://www.apa.org/practice/programs/dmhi/research-information/informed-consent-checklist

Balkin, R., & Juhnke, G. (2018). *Assessment in counseling: Practice and application.* Oxford University Press.

Berghuis, D. J., & Jongsma, A. E. J. (2014). *The adult psychotherapy progress notes planner.*

CAMs Care Preventing Suicide. (2021). *Home page.* https://cams-care.com/

Centers for Disease Control and Prevention. (2018). *Health Insurance Portability and Accountability Act of 1996 (HIPAA).* https://www.cdc.gov/phlp/publications/topic/hipaa.html#:~:text=The%20Health%20Insurance%20Portability%20and,the%20patient's%20consent%20or%20knowledge

Chen, J., & Benusa, A. (2017). HIPAA security compliance challenges: The case for small healthcare providers. *International Journal of Healthcare Management, 10*(2), 135–146. https://doi.org/10.1080/20479700.2016.1270875

CPH & Associates. (2007). Consent to treat minor (sole and joint legal custody) [Blog post]. *Avoiding Liability.* https://www.cphins.com/consent-to-treat-minor-sole-and-joint-legal-custody/

Gilbertson, J. (2020). *Telemental health: The essential guide to providing successful online therapy.* PESI.

Healthcare Providers Service Organization. (2021). *Risk management considerations in telehealth and telemedicine.* https://www.hpso.com/risk-education/individuals/articles/Risk-Management-Considerations-in-Telehealth-and-Telemedicine

Hodges, S. (2021). *The counseling practicum and internship manual: A resource for graduate counseling students (3rd ed.).* Springer Publishing Company.

Jaffee v. Redmond, 518 U.S.1. (1996). https://www.law.cornell.edu/supct/html/95-266.ZO.html

Lawley, J. (2012). HIPAA, HITECH and the practice counselor: Electronic records and practice guidelines. *The Professional Counselor, 2*(3), 192–200.

Luxton, D., Nelson, E., & Maheu, M. (2016). *A practitioner's guide to telemental health: How to conduct legal, ethical, and evidence-based telepractice.* American Psychological Association. https://doi.org/10.1037/14938-002

National Board for Certified Counselors. (2016). *NBCC policy regarding the provision of distance professional services.* https://www.nbcc.org/Assets/Ethics/NBCCPolicyRegardingPracticeofDistanceCounselingBoard.pdf

National Institute of Mental Health. (n.d.). *What is telemental health?* https://www.nimh.nih.gov/sites/default/files/documents/21-MH-8155-Telemental-Health.pdf

Novoa-Gomez, M., Pulido-Castelblanco, D., & Munoz-Martinez, A. (2020). Assessing the utility of the clinical behavioral case conceptualization categories: A contextual behavioral based formula model. *Journal of Contextual Behavioral Science, 18*, 53–58. https://doi.org/10.1016/j.jcbs.2020.08.055

Ramirez, H., Springmeyer, A., Weis, K., Espiritu, R., Wolf-Prusan, L., DeCelle, K., Heitkamp, T., & Clarke, B. (2020). *Telehealth clinical and technical considerations for mental health providers.* https://cars-rp.org/_MHTTC/docs/Telehealth%20Clinical%20Considerations.pdf

Remley, T., Herlihy, B., & Herlihy, S. (1997). The U.S. Supreme Court decision in *Jaffee v. Redmond*: Implications for counselors. *Journal of Counseling and Development, 75*(3), 213–218.

Sperry, L., Carlson, J., Duba, S. J., & Sperry, J. (Eds.). (2014). *Psychopathology and psychotherapy: DSM-5 diagnosis, case conceptualization, and treatment.* Taylor & Francis.

Suicide Prevention Resource Center. (2017). Collaborative assessment and management of suicidality (CAMS). https://www.sprc.org/resources-programs/collaborative-assessment-management-suicidality-cams

U.S. Department of Health and Human Services. (2013, January 25). *Business associate contracts.* https://www.hhs.gov/hipaa/for-professionals/covered-entities/sample-business-associate-agreement-provisions/index.html

Wheeler, A. M., & Bertram, B. (2019). *The counselor and the law: A guide to legal and ethical practice.* American Counseling Association.

Zubernis, L. D. S., & Snyder, M. J. (2015). *Case conceptualization and effective interventions: Assessing and treating mental, emotional, and behavioral disorders.* SAGE.

Credits

CHAPTER 7

Application of Telemental Health, Part 1

Young Children

Jen Green

It is in playing, and only in playing, that the individual child or adult is able to be creative and to use the whole personality, and it is only in being creative that the individual discovers the self.

–D. W. Winnicott, British pediatrician, 1896–1971

Learning Objectives

After reading this chapter, you should be able to do the following:

1. Identify effective models of telehealth when working with young children
2. Review developmentally appropriate activities that can be used during a telemental health session
3. Reflect on the pros and cons of telemental health with young children
4. Follow through with the provided personal reflection activities in preparation for providing telemental health services

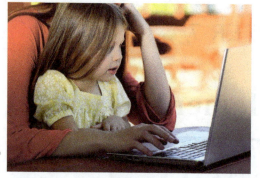

Image 7.1

Introduction

In February 2020, I returned from a Florida conference center having walked across the stage in celebration of completing my PhD. Joining me in celebrating were several hundred other participants completing their degrees and pridefully walking across the stage to receive the earned diploma with families and friends cheering us on! By March 2020, the local and national news had articulated the need for safety and precaution due to a harmful virus called coronavirus disease, COVID-19. Weeks after this breaking news, drastic changes began to unfold both personally and professionally. While the counseling field had been advocating for telehealth for many years, suddenly the term *telehealth* became well known to the general community within a few short weeks. State and federal mandates directed persons to "shelter in place," which became the norm for many across the United States and around the world. Schools, businesses, and families quickly followed new protocols, changing routines and schedules (Tolou-Shams et al., 2021). As a counselor with a focused practice working with young children and families, this mandate greatly impacted my professional work. One informative email directed me to no longer provide developmental services in homes; instead, I was quickly calling families to schedule telemental health services for the next several months.

I had trained for this position as an infant developmental specialist-counselor for over 20 years but still felt eager and anxious, like a horse jockeying for a position at the horse races. I was aware of telehealth services, but as many clinicians experienced (including myself), prior to the COVID-19 health crisis there was little to no training on telehealth services for this underserved population (Tolou-Shams et al., 2021). Thankfully, being a professional counselor, my training did emphasize the need to be flexible, rise to challenges, and always seek growth opportunities. Thus began a new adventure of providing services on this new platform to children and families. In preparation, I reviewed various telehealth modalities, explored age-appropriate developmental activities, and followed groups on social media who had been working in the field of telemental health long before the shelter-in-place mandates. This chapter is a small glimpse of my journey of providing telehealth services to young children and families. Before we begin, it is important to know that I will use the terms *telehealth* and *telemental health services* interchangeably. I have heard both terms used as I embarked on this new platform of providing services. For the purpose of this chapter, I define young children as ages from birth to 6, which has been my professional work experience with this age group. It is an exciting time to be a master's-level student obtaining a degree in the helping profession! We will begin examining the considerations of telehealth services for young children by exploring child development, ethical, moral, and legal factors, platform considerations, parent coaching, and age-appropriate activities.

CASE EXAMPLE

Brody is a 20-month-old child. The parents have contacted you because they are concerned about Brody's social interactions. Since the COVID-19 pandemic, Brody has been home with the parents. Due to state mandates, fear about the virus, and limited financial resources, the parents decided it was best for their family to stay home as much as possible. Each parent had a career that allowed each of them to work from home. Although the parents expressed it was a challenge to find a new work-home routine, they are thankful to have the opportunity to work from home. However, as Brody has aged over the months, the parents are concerned about his socioemotional development and are unsure how to best go about engaging Brody with social interactions. They tried to take him to the grocery store but noticed he started crying as they walked down the first food aisle. They have also tried to take him to a local park, but he clings to them and will not get down, also resulting in crying. The family would like to participate in telemental health services because they are not ready for in-person services and would like to know if there is a concern with Brody's development and what they can do about his crying when they do take him to the store or park.

Spend some time reflecting on how you would start telemental health services for this family. What would you like to observe from Brody? From the family? What do you need to consider when starting telemental health services with this family?

Child Development: A Brief Refresher

As a master's-level student, it is important to review life span development while working in the helping profession. Knowledge and understanding of development are helpful during the counseling process and treatment planning with all individuals, but especially when providing services to young children and families (Lamprecht & Sneha, 2018; Smith-Adcock & Tucker, 2017). For instance, when providing telehealth services, knowledge of child development may increase counselor self-efficacy and decrease frustration for the child, family, and you as a professional (Zandt & Barrett, 2017). Having knowledge and understanding of what is typical in development will help you as a clinician assess when development is uncharacteristic at various stages of development. I will be sharing a brief review of child development in this chapter, but a detailed examination of development can be located in any child development textbook or on the Zero to Three website (https://www.zerotothree.org/).

I believe each child is unique and constructs their own learning based on relationships and experiences. During your training, developmental theory will be discussed at length, so I will not go into great detail here in this chapter. However, I do regard Bronfenbrenner's ecological theory (Bronfenbrenner, 1986), which suggests a child's development is impacted by environmental experiences and opportunities. Theorists such as Kohlberg, Piaget, Vygotsky, Erikson, and Loevinger also propose theories describing child development. The book *A Therapist's Guide to Child Development: The Extraordinarily Normal Years*, edited by Dee C. Ray (2016), provides an outstanding summary of each theorist. I recommend reading this book at some point during your training and career. It provides an excellent overview of child development, which will aid in the understanding of telemental health with young children.

My work as an infant developmental specialist has provided years of observation of children's development among thousands of children and families of numerous backgrounds and cultures. I must share here that prior to obtaining a mental health counseling degree I began my professional career as a special education teacher and hold a bachelor's degree in elementary education and my first master's degree in special education. This background certainly has been beneficial while working in the field of mental health counseling. As a trainee, you may also have other degrees and knowledge in other careers, or are a parent, caregiver, or grandparent. These experiences provide a background of knowledge equally beneficial to the helping professions. In this chapter, I will focus on children ages 6 and younger, as this is my clinical expertise, and I invite you to continue researching this area for further information.

Let's get back to child development. Generally speaking, a baby begins social cues and connections during fetal development (Lickliter, 2011; Ray, 2016). While in the womb, the baby hears familiar voices and feels the sway and movement of a mother's walk (Joanna et al., 2018; Lickliter, 2011; Ray, 2016). Brain development occurs within the womb, but also after birth the new smells and sounds continue infiltrating the brain (Lickliter, 2011; Maya et al., n.d.). The baby quickly becomes familiar with parents and the natural

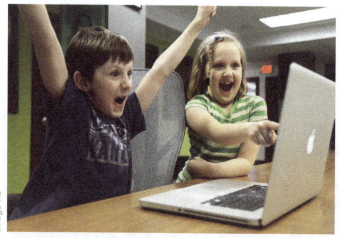

environment, and the bond between parent and child takes root (Maya et al., n.d.). Attachment and socio-emotional development immediately envelop like a matrix system circulating and filing its data for future use. Erikson identifies these beginning experiences as the stage of trust and mistrust (Smith-Adcock & Tucker, 2017).

Image 7.2

Birth to 3

Children from birth to 3 are learning many new skill sets. Gross motor skills, also known as large muscle movements, may include rolling, crawling, walking, climbing, jumping, hopping, and galloping (Ray, 2016). Language development for children during the first 3 years begins with cooing and babbling, progressing toward the production of consonant sounds and eventually words and full sentences (Ray, 2016).

In my professional experiences, hearing, cognitive development, and gross motor skills impact the development of language. Children at this age begin to develop an understanding of body parts, animal sounds, pictures, and objects. They may be learning how to drink from a bottle, cup, and straw and how to eat using fingers and a spoon. Zero to Three (n.d.) offers a free video that provides a summary of the development during the 1st year and articulates the importance of engaging with a child.

Three to 6

During the preschool years, one area of focus in development is socioemotional growth. Children are learning to share, take turns, follow rules to games, and follow routines (Ray, 2016). They may be more expressive in their emotions with the advancement of verbal words such as *scared*, *angry*, or *excited*. Friendships form, collaborative play evolves, and insecurity or anxious behaviors such as nail biting may be observed (Ray, 2016). As cognitive skills advance, children become aware of making moral decisions. Pretend play is one-way children learn how to make decisions, engage and understand conflict, and process feelings.

TIME TO BOOKMARK!

The National Association for the Education of Young Children offers events and topics providing parents and professionals resources and information on child development: https://www.naeyc. org/resources/topics.

Prior to graduating and thereafter, spend some time attending a conference, listening to a podcast, reading a book, or interviewing other professions about the ages and stages of child development. Membership to professional associations is also a valuable resource for clinicians. Telemental health with young children requires the knowledge and understanding of child development. Furthermore, individuals serving in the helping profession must also be aware of ethical, legal, and moral considerations.

Ethical and Legal Factors

Chapter 2 was dedicated to ethical and legal considerations for telemental health services; therefore, I will not go into detail on this topic here. Please review Chapter 2, this volume, for additional details on issues pertaining to legal and ethical considerations. However, I do believe it is important to address a few ethical and legal factors in this chapter that are particularly salient for working with young children and families. Consider the following questions to ask yourself prior to any telemental health session:

- Are the platform considerations HIPAA compliant?
- Have I disclosed to the family the strengths and barriers of telemental health?
- Am I prepared to offer brief technical support to guide the family should the platform selected stop working?
- Do I have an alternative method to contact the family when this occurs?

These questions can provide guidance when proactively considering dilemmas that may be encountered. In my own professional experience, I reflected on these questions while also thinking about what platforms to use for telemental health. Choosing a platform may be an individual choice; however, the employer or organization may also specifically direct you on which platform to use. In either case, it is important to understand the pros and cons of the platform selected. Additional resources, information, events, and membership options can be located at the American Telemedicine Association (ATA, https://www.americantelemed.org/).

Platform Considerations

In my situation, when the pandemic forced a drastic change in my work, I had to ask myself, "What platform is available to families and HIPAA compliant?" In the weeks ahead, my organization (based in California) sent an email indicating platforms the California Department of Human Services (CDHS, n.d.) identified as approved for developmental services. In my experience, Zoom for health care has been a priority for most families and the platform many families have chosen. Zoom is easily accessed, videoconferencing is available, and shared-screen time provides an opportunity for children to participate in the session. Zoom also offers a tab called "Whiteboard," which I have found helpful when I want to write and participate in the children's writing.

I have listed other platform considerations that are HIPAA compliant according to the Substance Abuse and Mental Health Services Administration (SAMHSA, n.d.). Prior to choosing a platform, consider if it can be accessed by the family, their degree of understanding, and if a contract is required by the provider. At the time of this writing, the Pacific Southwest Mental Health Technology Transfer Center, which is part of SAMHSA, identifies the following platforms:

- Doxy.me
- Updox
- Google G Suite/Hangouts Meet
- Vsee
- Skype for Business
- Zoom Healthcare

Parent Coaching

After selecting a platform, become familiar with approaches that can be easily utilized online. When working with young children and families, I follow a parent-coaching model. The general term *parent coaching* is defined by Kemp and Turnbull (2014):

> An adult learning strategy in which the coach promotes the learner's ability to reflect on his or her actions as a means to determine the effectiveness of an action or practice and develop a plan for refinement and use of the action in immediate and future situations. (p. 307)

Using this model, many strategies can be implemented when providing telehealth services. For example, I often engage in a conversation with the caregiver regarding any changes in development and behaviors observed at home from the caregiver's perspective. Parent coaching also provides me as a provider an opportunity to observe the child in the natural environment. For example, I will ask parents if they are willing and able to turn the video screen around onto the child playing or when they as the caregiver engage in play with the child. This observation time then provides me as the provider an opportunity to demonstrate skills and provide direct teaching to the caregiver. Kemp and Turnbull (2014) identify additional strategies to use in parent coaching such as offering guided practice, providing feedback, modeling or joint interaction, and problem solving. I support these additional strategies and have used each during telemental health sessions.

When a caregiver encounters a challenging behavior, it is helpful to observe the behavior. Therefore, I will ask the parent to spend a few minutes playing with their child and point out the behavior needing to be addressed. I can observe, provide feedback, and offer guided practice as the parent and child play. Observation can be applied when working with babies as well. I ask the caregiver to engage in play with the baby in what would be considered a normal routine at home: on the floor doing tummy time, in a highchair, or holding the baby on a lap. The caregiver will turn the camera for my observation and then talk, sing, or play with the baby while I observe, provide feedback, and guide the parent in newly directed social engagements. It is important to remember as a clinician to pay attention to nonverbal body language of the baby and the parent. This nonverbal language offers information such as "Is the baby done with this play? Bored? Tired? Is the tone of voice of the caregiver stimulating to the baby? Is the caregiver distracted, nervous, anxious, comfortable when the baby responds differently than expected by the caregiver? Do I as a clinician observe a connection between child and parent? What strengths do I as a clinician see between child and parent?" I always point out these strengths to the parent because my bias (which I encourage for all counselors!) is toward a strengths-based approach to parent coaching. Once I notice the parent and the child need a break, I spend some time talking to the parent again, offering new activities and available resources. In some instances, self-care and mindfulness strategies may be explored with the parent.

This general parent-coaching model is one that is similar to basic counseling skills. Parent–child interaction therapy (PCIT) and the gestalt parent-coaching model are two other parent-coaching modalities used in telehealth services for young children and families. These evidence-based approaches provide additional therapeutic techniques and strategies. Given the limited training of working with young children, having additional knowledge of techniques and strategies can be helpful for increasing counselor self-efficacy.

PCIT is an evidence-based approach that can be used with families and children aged 2 to 7. It is considered a short-term approach supporting parent–child interactions (Gurwitch et al., 2020). PCIT offers caregivers an opportunity to learn new strategies for challenging behaviors. This interactive format is home based. It allows for observation and collaboration between clinician and caregiver (Gurwitch et al., 2020). This approach is an option for telemental health services due to its versatility and flexibility.

The gestalt parent-coaching model is yet another telemental health model. This new approach supports building a supportive clinician–parent therapeutic relationship (Melnick, 2014). It is a strengths-based approach encouraging observation from the natural environment (Melnick, 2014). The gestalt parent-coaching model is based on the work of Gregory Bateson, who emphasizes the importance of focusing on what is working instead of what is not (Melnick, 2014). Based on general systems theory, this approach supports the process of building a trusting therapeutic relationship, increasing awareness of new parenting experiences, as well as integrating and providing exercises to mobilize new parenting experiences (Melnick, 2014).

Telemental health services can be a beneficial and collaborative means of providing services to young children and families (Gloff et al., 2015). By having an evidenced-based approach as a foundation to start telehealth services, the experience for the child, family, and clinician can be highly rewarding. When I work with families and young children using the telemental health format, it is my hope for the family to feel supported and encouraged and to create a nonjudgmental space for growth and learning to occur. My approach has been influenced by the person-centered approach identified by Carl Rogers. When I provide age-appropriate activities, I focus on the child's development and the family's goals for their child and the family system.

A SAMPLE OF MY GO-TO SOURCES

Agassi, M. (1996). *Hands are not for hitting.* Free Spirit Publishing.

American Association for Marriage and Family Therapy. (n.d.). *Home page.* https://aamft.org/

American Counseling Association. (n.d.). *Home page.* https://www.counseling.org/

American Psychological Association (n.d.). *Telepsychology best practices 101.* https://www.apa.org/career-development/telepsychology

Association for Play Therapy. (n.d.). *Home page.* https://www.a4pt.org/

Gates, M. (2016). *Good morning yoga.* Sounds True, Inc.

The National Association for the Education of Young Children. *Topics.* https://www.naeyc.org/resources/topics

The National Child Traumatic Stress Network. (n.d.). *Psychological first aid.* https://learn.nctsn.org/course/index.php?categoryid=11

Oaklander, V. (1989). *Window to our children.* Gestalt Journal Press.

Rowland, J. (2017). *The memory box: A book about grief.* Sparkhouse Family.

Verdick, E. (2010). *Calm-down time.* Free Spirit Publishing.

Yack, E., Aquilla, P., & Sutton, S., (2002). *Building bridges through sensory integration: Therapy for children with autism and other pervasive developmental disorders* (2nd ed). Future Horizons, Inc.

Zero to Three. (n.d.). *Home page.* https://www.zerotothree.org/

Examples of Age-Appropriate Activities in Telemental Health

In this section I share a few activities I have used during my telehealth sessions with young children and families. I too had to adapt ideas from books, browse social media groups, and ask other professionals what worked during their telehealth sessions as I delved into telemental health. I hope these ideas provide a sense of excitement for the work in this profession as you continue your research in telemental health for young children.

1. **Interactive observation**

    Encourage the parent to hold the baby or play with the baby on the floor or couch using a mat/blanket. Ask the parent to sing a song to the baby, talk to the baby, or play with the baby using their favorite toys. Observe the eye contact between parent and baby and the parent's tone of voice. Did the parent–child seem connected? Did the baby sustain eye contact? Notice the baby's body language and attention to the parent's body language. Did the baby kick legs or move arms with excitement? Did the parent seem comfortable engaging with the baby? Identify sounds within the environment that may be distracting, reinforcing, overwhelming, or underwhelming. Talk to the parent about your observations and point out strengths you notice. Ask the parent to discuss their own observations and concerns, and then provide new recommendations or suggestions supporting parent growth or a child's development.

2. **Bibliotherapy** (here are a few examples I use in my practice)

   a. *Calm-Down Time* by Elizabeth Verdick. On screen, read the book with toddlers or preschool-aged children and the caregiver. After reading the book, practice deep breathing techniques with the child and caregiver. I like to use the "five-finger breathing" technique, which can be located on general social media sites. Take the index finger on one hand, draw it up the thumb of the other hand, and breathe in. Bring the index finger down the thumb and breathe out. Draw the finger up the pointer finger of the hand and breathe in, bring it down, breath out, and so forth until breathing in and out has been completed on each finger. This activity can be repeated until the child or parent feels calm. It can be used safely in most natural environments.

   b. *Hands Are Not for Hitting* by Martine Agassi. Encourage the parent and child to sit in a comfortable location such as a bean bag chair, the couch, or cuddled in a blanket. On screen read this book to the parent and child. After reading the book, sing a clapping song with the child and parent, modeling appropriate use for the hands when having a big feeling such as anger or frustration. I often make songs up at the moment. You can try this too. Make up a song about feeling frustrated or angry to show that clapping hands is what to do instead of hitting or throwing. One popular toddler-preschool nursery rhyme is *Open Shut Them*. This rhythmic tune is a way parents can redirect assertive behavior, reminding children what to do with hands when having "big" emotions. When I work with families, I always like to emphasize saying this slowly, connecting with eye contact and a calm tone, and modeling the hand gestures.

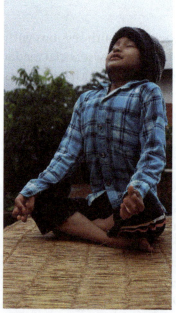

Image 7.3

Open Shut Them
Open, shut them (open hands, close hands)
Open, shut them (open hands, close hands)
Give a little clap (clap hands)
Open, shut them (open hands, close hands)
Open, shut them (open hands, close hands)
Fold them in your lap (fold hands in lap)

   c. *Good Morning Yoga* by Mariam Gates. Read this book with the child or child and parent providing a colorful illustration of yoga poses that can provide a sense of peace and calmness. As a clinician, practice these poses during the telehealth session with the child. Explore visualization strategies with the child if the child has the cognitive understanding of this concept. If you are working with a younger child, such as a preschool-aged child, encourage the parent and child to walk through the natural environment collecting objects to create a "cool-down box" such as a coloring book, a book, a slinky, a stuffed animal, or a Koosh ball.

   d. *The Memory Box* by Joanna Rowland. Losing a loved one can be difficult for children. Grief, though, can also occur when there is a change in routine, a loss of attending school, loss of a pet, or a loss of being around friends and family. Prior to the telehealth session, ask the parent to provide a box, crayons, markers, stickers, pictures, glue, and tape. These items can be used to decorate the memory box. As the child decorates the box, the child can share stories or details of what will go inside the box. Basic counseling skills can provide a safe space for the child to process grief. As a clinician, spend time with the parent, providing resources and extended activities to do at home with the child.

3. **Play-Doh**

   If the child is able and the parent is willing, spend some time playing with Play-Doh, kinetic sand, or thera-putty together. While engaging with this hands-on activity, talk to the parent about redirection and sensory play, which can de-escalate "big" feelings a child may experience. If you are unfamiliar with sensory play or sensory processing, talk to an occupational therapist, read a book, and/or attend training to begin gaining a better understanding of this term and its importance in development. This is especially important for a child who may have a developmental diagnosis.

4. **Bubble bubble pop**

   Prior to the telehealth session, contact the parent and invite them to have a bottle of bubbles ready for the session. This can be a time to talk about happy feelings, sad feelings, big feelings, and little feelings. Remind the child that feelings also come and go just as the bubble does when it pops. As you blow bubbles together, encourage the parent to also share the "themed" feelings. End the session by drawing a bubble, or many bubbles on a piece of paper using crayons, markers, and colored pencils. Zoom has a tab called "Whiteboard," which is an excellent tool to use for participating with the child. You can draw your own bubble, and children and parents together can label feelings or events in the bubble(s).

Provide a homework activity for the family to work on until the next session. This could be a repeat of the bubble play or a mindfulness activity.

5. **Animal walks**

Children need to stay active. This sensory activity can provide input into the hands, feet, and body, which may help build body awareness and calm an over-whelmed, anxious child. Here are a few examples of animal walks that can be fun to do during telehealth sessions: bunny hop, frog jumps, bear walk, crab crawl, turtle crouch, seal walk. As a clinician, print out pictures for the child as a reminder of the animal walks practiced, or create a PowerPoint of the animal walks that can be accessed from home for the parent and child to do together.

6. **Family scavenger hunt Bingo**

By creating a sense of teamwork, scavenger hunts can provide an opportunity for families to work together. This game can also provide you as a clinician an opportunity to observe the interactions between family members. It also allows families to discuss topics such as what makes the family feel safe, something the family likes to do together, a favorite toy, or something unique to the family.

7. **Sensory bags/bins**

Sensory play is an outlet for the child to explore learning by using the senses such as taste, touch, smell, movement, or sound (Watts, 2020). Sensory play allows the brain to regulate emotions and foster learning connections (Watts, 2020). One idea for sensory play is using sensory bags or sensory bins. Using a gallon-sized baggie or smaller, fill the baggie with various textures such as hair gel, rice, beans, popcorn seeds, oatmeal, or anything else that may be available within the home. The child can squish the baggie using hands or feet, feeling the texture inside. As a caregiver or parent, provide language connections by describing the textures in one word to the child (soft, bumpy, etc.), or model deep breathing as the child plays with the sensory baggie, which can provide a sense of calmness. Shoebox-sized bins can be used with older children and those who no longer put small objects in the mouth. Similar to the baggie, fill a 6-quart bin with rice, beans, cereal, rocks, or any other textural item. Objects such as a spoon, car, small plastic animal, or other small toys can be placed in the bin for play. This can be helpful when a child is having a difficult time touching the texture. The object provides a safe barrier from touching a texture that feels unsafe, unfamiliar, and uncomfortable to the touch. A child diagnosed with autism, or a sensory processing disorder, may exhibit characteristics such as the one described. As a clinician, consulting with an occupational therapist can also be helpful when working with children with a developmental delay. Occupational therapists and speech therapists can offer additional sensory bin suggestions and strategies for using sensory bins/baggies when working with a child who may feel anxious, sad, or have sensory processing concerns and language delays.

8. **Simon Says**

This is a wonderful activity regulating emotions. A child who is agitated, unfocused, overwhelmed, or hyper may need the use of play to regain focus and a sense of calmness. Encourage the child or include the family to jump, dance, do jumping jacks or toe touches, or push the palm of their hands together to calm the active body. When playing this game, notice nonverbal cues that may show a calm body such as improved eye contact, decrease in rapid speech, improved attention span, a smile, or a decrease in hyper body movements. Use this activity throughout different times of the day, noticing if there is a change in behaviors after using the activity in the morning, afternoon, or evening. Perhaps the activity isn't helping the child and behaviors have escalated or increased; then it may be time to stop the activity and adjust the intervention to a different calming strategy. Remember, every child is unique!

9. **Drawing**

Prior to the telehealth session, ask the parent to have paper and writing utensils available. A variety works, particularly so the child has options (pencils, markers, crayons, highlighters). Provide simple prompts during the session: Draw a safe space, draw your favorite toy, draw yourself as your favorite animal, or draw yourself as a superhero. As a trainee, spend some time reviewing various approaches of play therapy when considering this drawing activity. Two possible considerations to explore in your efforts could be gestalt play therapy or Adlerian play therapy. While exploring the tenets of play therapy, consider asking how these play therapy philosophies are similar and how they differ. How does each play therapy approach view the importance of drawing when using this activity with a young child? What is my role as the therapist? What is the role of the child? How and in what ways is this therapeutic experience helping the young child regulate emotions and process "big" feelings?

10. **Games**

Games are a wonderful tool to engage children and teach important life skills such as turn taking, following rules, and good sportsmanship. Examples that can be adapted for telehealth sessions include Uno, Candyland, Bingo, Chutes and Ladders, or Jenga. Teachers Pay Teachers is a resource created by teachers but is available to all professionals. The resources available on this site can be purchased for a minimal fee. Candyland for telehealth sessions is one example (Teachers Pay Teachers, n.d.).

11. **Connection activities**

It is important for parents and children to connect, especially if stressful situations are occurring at home and in the child's world. These activities may be helpful for building connection: Rub lotion in their hands and trace the lines of the hands, encouraging the parent to talk about what they love about their child; paint each other nails, play "I Spy," imitate facial expressions in a mirror, feed each other foods such as Cheerios or M&M's, making eye contact and smiling together. The options here are limitless, and this is an excellent opportunity to bring families together in fun and creative ways!

Chapter Summary

Telemental health is a service that is now available throughout much of the world due to the pandemic crisis. It provides an opportunity for families living in rural communities to have access to mental health care and support for the child and family when limited resources are available in a community or changes in daily routines have occurred. In my experience thus far, families have voiced appreciation for the option of having in-person or telemental health services. When the child is ill, parents have articulated that having telehealth services available allows them to keep the appointment without feeling they have to cancel a session, thus maintaining the support needed during times of stress and crisis.

There are several telehealth platform options available. However, maintaining HIPAA compliance is critical when considering the options. In addition, it is important to become familiar with therapeutic models used for telehealth sessions. Parent coaching, PCIT, and gestalt parent coaching are a few evidence-based approaches. However, the Association for Play Therapy (n.d.), the American Counseling Association (ACA), and the American Association for Marriage and Family Therapy (AAMFT) can provide additional training and resources in the area of telemental health, treatment, and activities.

Prior to working with young children and families, aim to, if possible, start the initial session with a parent consultation first. Review the informed consent, talk about the pros and cons of using technology, set a plan to reconnect with the parent should you and the parent or child have technology glitches during the sessions, and establish a safe, trusting environment online with appropriate boundaries. Establishing appropriate and practical expectations creates a safe, trusting therapeutic relationship between clinician and family (Mellenthin, 2018).

By having a solid understanding of child development, a clinician providing telemental health services is familiar with typical development and development that may be uncustomary for the child's age. Training and knowledge in child development also establishes age-appropriate expectations in the home, the community, and even during telehealth sessions. Clinicians grounded in child development working with young children may notice an increase in counselor self-efficacy. When I believe I am capable of carrying out a task, I am more confident in my abilities and can draw on these strengths when providing encouragement and support to the parents who are learning strategies or activities to work with challenging behaviors at home.

Historically, key figures in the field of child development have reinforced and emphasized the critical need of play for optimal development. For example, Jean Piaget underscored in his career the importance of children playing things through in order to think things through (Howe, 1977). Virginia Axline stated, "Enter into children's play and you will find the place where their minds, hearts, and souls meet" (1974, p. 9). "Play helps us break free" expressed Eliana Gil (2015, p. 451). Utilizing telehealth services with young children and families means finding an alternative way to play, observe, and learn together.

APPLICATION ACTIVITIES

We covered quite a bit in this chapter, and you can use these prompts to further reflect on and journal on key themes addressed.

1. **Make a list of other professionals you may need to consult with while working with young children and families.**
   Why is it important to know about these other professionals, and how might they help your role as a clinician when working with young children and families? Think outside the realm of therapy when reflecting on this activity. For example, I work with many occupational therapists who aid in my understanding of sensory processing.

2. **Make a chart of each skill set for each stage of development (birth, infant, toddler, preschool, elementary).**
   Review development in each area of the following skill sets for each stage: cognitive, fine motor, gross motor, socioemotional, self-help/adaptive, expressive language, receptive language, nutrition, sleep patterns, sensory processing. What changes do you notice? Why might understanding child development be important for your role as a counselor?

3. **If you have social media, locate and join a group or organization that specializes in telemental health for children.**
   International groups may also be available on social media. Why is it important for a counselor to understand diversity and cultural considerations when using telemental health services for young children and families?

4. **Check with your state board to see if additional certification or training is required to work with young children.**

References

American Telemedicine Association. (n.d). *Home page.* https://www.americantelemed.org/

Axline, V. M. (1974). *Play therapy.* The Random House Publishing Group.

Bronfenbrenner, U. (1986). Ecology of the family as a context for human development: Research perspectives. *Developmental Psychology, 22* (6), 723–742.

California Department of Human Services. (n.d.). *Home page.* https://www.chhs.ca.gov/

Gil. E. (2015). *Play in family therapy* (2nd ed.). The Guilford Press.

Gloff, N. E., LeNoue, S. R., Novins, D. K., & Myers, K. (2015). Telemental health for children and adolescents. *International Review of Psychiatry, 27*(6), 513–524. https://doi-org/10.3109/09540261.2015.1086322

Gurwitch, R., Salem, H., Nelson, M., & Cornes, J. (2020). *Leveraging parent-child interaction therapy and telehealth capacities to address the unique needs of young children during the COVID-19 public health crisis.* American Psychological Association.

Howe, L. T. (1977). Jean Piaget's theory of cognitive development: an overview and appraisal. *Perkins Journal, 31*(1), 27–64.

Joanna, J. P., Robert, D., Kalpashri, K., Paul, M. M., Lonnie, Z., & Ronald, M. H. (2018). A description of externally recorded womb sounds in human subjects during gestation. *PLoS ONE, 13*(5), e0197045. https://doi.org/10.1371/journal.pone.0197045

Kemp, P., & Turnbull, A., (2014). Coaching with parents in early intervention: An interdisciplinary research synthesis. *Journal of Early Childhood Intervention, 27*(5), 305–324. https://doi.org/10.1097/IYC.0000000000000018

Lamprecht, L. M., & Sneha, P. M. (2018). Developing a pre-practicum environment for beginning counselors: Growing my counselor educator self. *Journal of Counselor Preparation and Supervision, 11*(2). https://digitalcommons.sacredheart.edu/jcps/vol11/iss2/3/

Lickliter, R. (2011). The integrated development of sensory organization. *Clinics in Perinatology, 38*(4), 591–603. https://doi.org/10.1016/j.clp.2011.08.007

Maya, O., Elizabeth, G., & Regina, S. (n.d.). Early life adversity during the infant sensitive period for attachment: Programming of behavioral neurobiology of threat processing and social behavior. *Developmental Cognitive Neuroscience, 25*, 145–159.

Mellenthin, C. (2018). *Play therapy: Engaging and powerful techniques for the treatment of childhood disorders.* PESI.

Melnick, H. (2014). Gestalt parent coaching: A new model for intervening in family systems. *Gestalt Review, 18*(2), 130–145.

Ray, D. (2016). *A therapist's guide to child development: The extraordinarily normal years.* Routledge.

Smith-Adcock, S., & Tucker, C. (2017). *Counseling children and adolescents: Connecting theory, development, and diversity.* SAGE.

Substance Abuse and Mental Health Services Association. (n.d.). *Home page.* https://www.samhsa.gov/

Teachers Pay Teachers. (n.d.). *Candy Land for telehealth.* https://www.teacherspayteachers.com/Product/Candy-Land-for-Telehealth-6273347

Tolou-Shams, M., Folk, J., Stuart, B., Mangurian, C., & Fortuno, L., (2021, June 10). Rapid creation of child telemental health services during COVID-19 to promote continued care for under-served children and families. *Psychological Services.* Advance online publication. http://dx.doi.org/10.1037/ser0000550

Watts, M. (2020). *Exciting sensory bins for curious kids: 60 easy creative play projects that boost brain development, calm anxiety and build fine motor skills.* Page Street Publishing.

Zandt, F., & Barrett, S. (2017). *Creative ways to help children manage big feelings: A therapist's guide to working with preschool and primary children.* Jessica Kingsley.

Zero to Three. (n.d.). *Early development: The first three years set the stage for lifelong success.* https://www.zerotothree.org/issue-areas/early-development/

CHAPTER 8

Application of Telemental Health, Part 2

Adolescents and Older Adults

Missy Fauser

We think we listen, but very rarely do we listen with real understanding, true empathy. Yet listening, of this very special kind, is one of the most potent forces for change that I know.

–Carl Rogers

Learning Objectives

After reading this chapter, you should be able to do the following:

1. Identify specific considerations for providing telemental health services to adolescent and older adult clients
2. Establish and maintain a therapeutic alliance in a telemental health setting with adolescent and older adult clients
3. Describe several evidence-based approaches to utilize when providing telemental health services to adolescent and older adult clients
4. Develop creative approaches to building rapport with adolescent and older adult clients

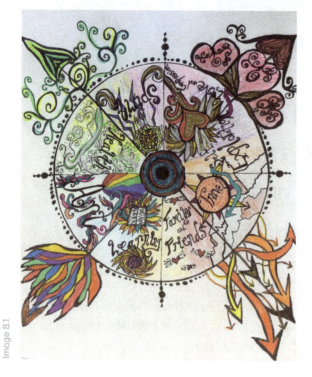

Image 8.1

Introduction

In this chapter, we will explore approaches, techniques, and considerations for providing telemental health (TMH) services to adolescents and older adults. Throughout my career, I have worked with many different age groups, but I continually find myself drawn to working with children, adolescents, and older adults. My background as an art therapist helps me to engage my clients through imagination and creativity. While there are many approaches and techniques to learn, I have chosen to discuss those that I utilize often and that are easily adaptable to the TMH session, including person-centered, mindfulness-based, cognitive behavioral , psychoeducation, and reminiscence therapy. While these techniques can be applied across different populations, this chapter will specifically apply them when considering TMH counseling with adolescents and older adults.

Providing Telemental Health Services to Adolescents

In a 2018 survey by Pew Research Center, 95% of adolescents aged 13–17 reported that they had access to a smartphone, and 45% reported that they are online "almost constantly." These statistics and other studies (Kenny et al., 2015; Nelson & Bui, 2010) suggest that adolescents have an inherent understanding and openness to utilizing the technological applications and platforms that are necessary for TMH services. TMH helps to provide services to adolescents

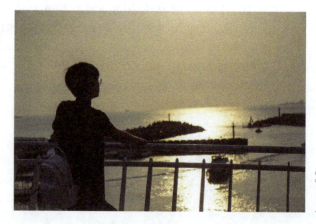

Image 8.2

and families living outside major metropolitan areas who tend to have difficulty in accessing evidence-based mental health interventions (Gloff et al., 2015). TMH also allows clinicians to provide services to adolescents in their natural settings such as their home (Comer & Myers, 2016; Gloff et al., 2015), schools (Comer & Myers, 2016; Stephan et al., 2016) and juvenile justice settings (Batastini, 2016). While there is a gap in the literature with regard to client satisfaction with TMH services, recent data suggests that adolescents, parents, and referring providers have reported high levels of satisfaction with TMH services (Egede et al., 2009; Goldstein & Glueck, 2016; Vander Stoep, 2017; Xie et al., 2013).

While there are many benefits to utilizing TMH with adolescents, there are also some concerns that distance counseling may result in a decrease of emotional connectedness with clients (Batastini, 2016). Another limitation is that access to technology may not be readily available to all youth, especially those who come from underprivileged or low socioeconomic backgrounds (Batastini, 2016; Comer & Myers, 2016; Jones et al., 2014). In addition, rural areas may lack the infrastructure for TMH services (Hage et al., 2013; Simms et al., 2011). It is also important to note that some information, such as behavioral cues that are outside of the camera frame, may be missed (Batastini, 2016). Despite these potential barriers, studies show that limitations appear to be less prevalent when providing TMH services to youth (Comer & Myers, 2016; Goldstein & Glueck, 2016).

Ethical Considerations When Counseling Adolescent Clients

Providing mental health services at a distance creates a need for additional ethical considerations. Telemedicine and mental health associations have discussed the importance of maintaining ethical best practice when providing TMH services to adolescent clients (American Academy of Child and Adolescent Psychiatry [AACAP] Committee on Telepsychiatry & AACAP Committee on Quality Issues, 2017; American Counseling Association [ACA], 2014, Section H.; American Psychological Association, 2013; American Telemedicine Association [ATA], 2017). The ATA (2017) has provided the following basic ethical considerations for working with children and adolescents:

a. Incorporate organizational values and ethics statements into the administrative policies and procedures for telemental health;
b. Be aware of medical and other professional discipline codes of ethics when using telemental health;
c. Inform the patient and parents of their rights and responsibilities when receiving care at a distance (through telemental health) including the right to refuse to use telemental health;

d. Provide patients, parents, and providers with a formal process for resolving ethical questions and issues that might arise as a result of a telemental health encounter; and

e. Eliminate any conflict of interest to influence decisions made about, for, or with patients who receive care via telemental health. Best ethical research practices shall also be followed in telemental health, as in all telemedicine settings. (p. 22)

TMH providers are encouraged to seek additional training and education, as well as seek out peer mentorship and clinical supervision with those who have experience in TMH "in order to maintain high quality care, facilitate therapeutic engagement, and produce positive outcomes" (ATA, 2017, p. 22). It is also important to be aware that legal and regulatory guidelines vary across states. The ATA (2017) states, "The provider shall practice within the jurisdictional policies and regulations for the treatment of youth with particular attention to the age of majority, consent to care, and mandated reporting. Special attention should focus on regulatory issues in the treatment of vulnerable youth, such as those in state custody" (p. 25). Although the informed consent is typically signed by the adolescent and the parents/guardians, the ACA (2014) code of ethics specifically indicates that clients such as adolescents are considered not legally eligible to give their voluntary informed consent, due to their minor status, but the documentation should be noted that the adolescent client still can sign and have the right to their personal protection of confidentiality.

Developing a Therapeutic Alliance With the Adolescent Client

As with any counseling relationship, building rapport is the first step to developing a therapeutic alliance with the client. A strong therapeutic alliance is associated with favorable treatment outcomes in youth (Cirasola et al., 2021; Karver et al., 2018) and is a common factor in efficacious therapies (Cirasola et al., 2021; Horvath, 2018). During the beginning of therapy, it is important to begin to build trust with the client (Goldstein & Glueck, 2016). Adolescents may require reassurance that their privacy and confidentiality will not be compromised, their sessions will not be recorded, and no one will be present in the session without the client's permission (ATA, 2017; Goldstein & Glueck, 2016).

The next step in developing a therapeutic alliance is allowing space for the client to share about themselves and "settle in" to the idea of therapy. Allowing the client space to share about the people and things that are important to them, such as family, friends, pets, and hobbies, is a great place to start. Finding creative ways to engage the client can also be helpful during this time. This might include encouraging them to utilize technology to share their favorite music, videos, artwork, or photographs during the TMH session (Goldstein & Glueck, 2016).

For most of my TMH sessions with adolescent clients, they contact me from their room. As I get to know them in the first session, I often ask them to take me on a tour of their room if they are comfortable with doing so, or to do a show-and-tell of items that are of importance for them. Much of an adolescent's personality can be seen through the items and decorations that are in their room. Specific items and artwork allow the adolescent the opportunity to share about themselves and allow me to ask them questions to get to know them better. I may also provide a few brief moments of self-disclosure if I see things that I connect with, which allows the client to get to know me a bit as well. I almost always see one or two items that I can connect with, such as a poster or character figurine. There are many similar ways to bring creativity into a TMH session with a client, and we will explore this further as we move into discussing theoretical approaches and techniques.

Theoretical Approaches and Techniques When Counseling Adolescents in TMH Settings

Research on evidence-based therapeutic approaches when providing TMH services with adolescents has increased as technology has advanced over the last 20 years (ATA, 2017; Gloff et al., 2015; Lau et al., 2021; Nelson & Patton, 2017). While several studies report positive outcomes for various approaches, much of the literature on TMH interventions with adolescents focuses on person-centered approaches (Goldstein & Glueck, 2016; Kemp et al., 2020), cognitive behavioral therapy (CBT; Himle et al., 2012; Spence et al., Goldstein 2006; Storch et al., 2011), and psychoeducation for parents and guardians (Bronstein et al., 2021; Chi & Demiris, 2015; Heitzman-Powell et al., 2013; Xie et al., 2013).

Person-Centered Therapy

It can be argued that the foundational skills in a contemporary person-centered approach are the foundational skills that every therapist needs to establish rapport, build a therapeutic alliance, and allow the client a safe space to share about their thoughts, emotions, and concerns (Goldstein & Glueck, 2016; Kemp et al., 2020). Adolescents often feel like they are not understood and that their thoughts and emotions are not validated. Conveying the person-centered elements of genuine empathy, unconditional positive regard, congruence, and nonjudgment allows the clinician to create a space free from everyday assumptions and demand, as well as provide the client with validation and understanding (Bryant-Jefferies et al., 2017).

One of my favorite TMH interventions to do with adolescents is called *Song of the Week*. Each week the client chooses a song to share with me. We listen to the song and then the client shares their thoughts about the song, such as what emotions it evokes in them, the meaning they find in the lyrics, and whether they connect with the musician's other work. If the client is up for it, we also each create a piece of art in response to the music and share it with each other.

Cognitive Behavioral Therapy

Findings from many studies have demonstrated that CBT interventions have positive outcomes with many adolescent populations, including those diagnosed with ADHD (Myers et al., 2015; Vander Stoep et al., 2017), tic disorders (Himle et al., 2012), obsessive compulsive disorder (OCD; Comer & Barlow, 2014; Storch et al., 2011), depression (Nelson et al., 2006; Reyes-Portillo et al., 2014), anxiety (Reyes-Portillo et al., 2014; Spence et al., 2006), autism (Oshima et al., 2020), and those who have experienced trauma (Jones et al., 2014). One way to easily adapt CBT to the TMH platform includes the use of handouts and homework. The clinician can email the handouts to the client ahead of time and then the completed handouts can be reviewed during the session or sent back to the clinician via secure email using photos or scans (Storch et al., 2011). If the client does not have access to a printer at home, the worksheets can be modified so that they can be filled out online or be printed by the clinician ahead of time and mailed to the client.

Some clinicians embrace technology fully by providing their adolescent clients with recommendations to access mobile phone apps (Chan et al., 2014; Kenny et al., 2015) and online CBT modules (Tillfors et al., 2011) with activities that can be completed by the client in between sessions for homework. At the time of this writing, Moodfit (Roble Ridge Software LLC, 2022) is one of the most popular mobile phone apps for mental health. The app has many uses, most notably CBT exercises, mood and gratitude journals, and guided breathing exercises. It also has standardized self-rating mental health assessments, such as the PHQ-9 (Kroenke et al., 2001) and GAD-7 (Kroenke et al., 2006), that can be completed by clients and shared with the clinician to help track symptoms over time (Roble Ridge Software LLC, 2022). Other apps, such as Bearable (Bearable LTD, 2022) can also help clients track their mood and symptoms, which in turn helps them increase self-awareness and provide a better overview of their well-being to doctors and therapists. The utilization of this technology in between sessions can also help provide extra support for clients, especially in instances where weekly sessions are not possible.

Psychoeducation for Parents and Guardians

As mentioned earlier, including the parents and guardians in treatment is an important consideration when working with adolescents. This might include psychoeducation to increase parent and guardian knowledge and awareness of the client's diagnosis, which in turn helps to decrease stigma and increase self-awareness (Oshima et al., 2020). It might also include teaching coping skills and behavioral strategies that will help parents and guardians learn how to best support their child (Heitzman-Powell et al., 2013; Reese et al., 2013; Xie et al., 2013), as well as learn how to manage their own emotions and stress (Gümüs et al., 2020; Krysinska et al., 2020).

I offer TMH psychoeducation consultations to all the parents and guardians of my adolescent clients. I let my clients know about these meetings before I have them and share with them the purpose of the meeting and the information I will be providing to their parents and guardians. I find these consultations to be especially helpful when I am working with a client who has experienced trauma. Often parents and guardians have a difficult time understanding the symptoms and behaviors of their child following a traumatic experience. I utilize slideshows over the video conferencing platform to provide information on the common thoughts, feelings, and behaviors that often occur in people who have experienced trauma, the body's response to a traumatic event, common triggers, and helpful coping skills. The consultation also provides parents and guardians the space to ask any questions they may have regarding trauma and treatment approaches. I follow up the meetings via email to provide informational worksheets to the parents to have for future reference.

There are many useful tools and resources you can use with adolescent clients to support them in identifying their thoughts, feelings, and behaviors. One worksheet I have found particularly useful in working with both teens and parents is provided by the University of Michigan (2013) in their online Trails to Wellness program. You can find many resources on their website.

TIME TO BOOKMARK!

University of Michigan: https://www.trailstowellness.org/

Some of the most helpful personal characteristics I have discovered over my many years of working with adolescents is the importance of honesty, flexibility, humor, and creativity. The feedback I get from many adolescents regarding the helpfulness of therapy is that it is a relief for them to have an adult in their life who truly listens to their concerns without judgment or condescension. It is easy for adults to forget what it is like to be a teenager, and they will say things such as "It's not that big of a deal," "Just get over it," or "Wait until you're older; then you will know what real problems are." Imagine how invalidating that can be! As therapists, we have the opportunity to provide validation and understanding to someone who often feels misunderstood. I find this is not only true for adolescents, but for older adults as well. We will explore this more as we move into the next section of the chapter, which will discuss considerations, approaches, and techniques for providing TMH services to older adult clients.

Providing Telemental Health Services With Older Adult Clients

In 2021, the Pew Research Center surveyed adults ages 65 and older. They discovered that 64% of these adults reported that they had a broadband connection at home, and 61% reported that they own a smartphone (Pew Research Center, 2021). The increased use of internet and smartphones among this age group suggests that they are growing more comfortable with utilizing technology, including the various applications and videoconferencing platforms that are required for TMH sessions.

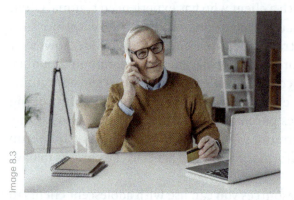

Image 8.3

Older adult clients often struggle with reduced mobility and lack of access to reliable transportation; thus, TMH is a helpful alternative. TMH services increase the potential for treatment adherence and outcomes while helping to maintain the safety of older adult clients (Egede et al., 2009; Pruit et al., 2014). This is especially true for clients who live in rural areas (Egede et al., 2009; Jones et al., 2014). TMH also has the potential to reduce the stigma many clients associate with traditional mental health care (Egede et al., 2009).

Another benefit of TMH services is that it supports the concept of allowing older adults to "age in place" (Wang et al., 2019). The goal of "aging in place" is to enable people to live their preferred lifestyle in familiar surroundings, allowing them to avoid residential care (Boldy et al., 2011; Peek et al., 2019). This in turn helps to promote a higher quality of life, which is an important aspect in the mental health and well-being of older adult clients (Kuziemsky et al., 2020; Peek et al., 2019).

Some older adults may not feel comfortable with the technology required to engage in TMH services, and they may encounter difficulties due to visual and hearing impairments (Shang et al., 2020). It is important to ensure that an older adult client's knowledge of technology is taken into consideration (Peek et al., 2019). Current telehealth and TMH systems tend to require older adults to adapt to the technology rather than the technology fitting the context of the individual (Peek et al., 2019). Research findings also suggest that TMH services are not suitable for older adults who are emotionally unstable, impulsive, or have poor coping skills, and those suffering from dementia or paranoia (Shang et al., 2020).

Ethical Considerations When Counseling Older Adults

When working with older adult clients, it is often important to collaborate with their family and service providers, such as their doctors and case managers, especially when a client is unable to be assessed in person (Kuziemsky et al., 2020; Yang et al., 2009). While collaborating with others, a counselor must maintain the privacy and confidentiality of their clients. Before discussing the case with family members and other service providers, a release of information (ROI) must be obtained (ACA, 2014; Yang et al., 2009). Some elderly clients will have a court-appointed guardian. According to the American Bar Association's Commission on Law and Aging (2006), a guardian is "a person who has qualified as a guardian of an incapacitated person pursuant to appointment by the court" (p. 40). If the client has a court-appointed guardian, the guardian will need to provide consent before TMH services can begin.

Another consideration when working with older adults is the need to balance respect for client autonomy with beneficence. Clinicians who work with older adults often experience "a tension between their desire to support the rights of patients to make the decisions that govern their lives and their investment in promoting patient welfare when patients' decisions appear to be inconsistent with their welfare" (Bush et al., 2017, p. 35). This decision can become even more complex when the decision-making capacity of an older adult client is in question (Bush et al., 2017). During these times, collaboration with the client and the client's family and other service providers can aid the counselor in deciding the best course of action (Bush et al., 2017; Kuziemsky et al., 2020).

An additional responsibility in promoting client welfare includes mandatory reporting. Counselors are ethically and legally obligated to report the mistreatment of vulnerable populations, including older adults (Bush et al., 2017). The National Adult Protective Services Association (NAPSA, 2018) identifies three forms of mistreatment of the elderly, including abuse, neglect, and exploitation. Abuse is defined as the intentional infliction of harm onto a person that can be perpetrated either sexually, physically, verbally, or emotionally (NAPSA, 2018). Neglect is a form of mistreatment by individuals resulting from inadequate attention, especially through carelessness or disregard for the needs of others (NAPSA, 2018). Financial exploitation occurs when a person misuses or takes the assets of a vulnerable adult for their own personal benefit. This frequently occurs without the explicit knowledge or consent of a senior or disabled adult, depriving them of vital financial resources for their personal needs (NAPSA, 2018). State laws govern the protection and reporting requirements of older adults, and investigations are enforced through state adult protective service agencies (Forman & McBride, 2010; NAPSA, 2018).

While the ethical considerations discussed in this chapter may seem overwhelming if you are just starting out as a counselor-in-training, keep in mind that your future fieldwork site/workplace will have specific procedures to follow when these situations arise. In addition, each state has their own procedure for the reporting of suspected mistreatment and abuse of vulnerable populations, including available resources to walk you through the process. It is also important to remember that you will have the support of clinical supervisors and consultation with colleagues to help you along the way.

Developing a Therapeutic Alliance With Older Adults

The importance of building rapport and developing a strong therapeutic alliance was discussed earlier in the chapter. With regard to building rapport with older adults, simply asking them about themselves, their families, and their pets is a good way to get started (Yang et al., 2009). Many older adult clients are open to sharing their many life experiences, and they typically enjoy getting the chance to talk to someone because they often feel lonely, especially if they live independently and alone (Kampfe, 2015; Yang et al., 2009). Using video platforms or HIPPA-compliant email/chat features is a great opportunity to encourage them to share photos of themselves and their families, as well as items such as cards and gifts from loved ones. This is helpful in building rapport and strengthening the therapeutic alliance, while also gathering important information on your client. It is also important to assure older adults that their privacy will be respected and that they will be notified if the clinician feels that their family or doctors need to know any information about the client before the information is shared (Kampfe, 2015). This helps to establish trust and collaboration with the client and their care team.

My favorite way to build rapport and continue a therapeutic alliance with an older adult client includes having them share photos of themselves, their families, and friends throughout the years. I often connect with my clients over a love of traveling, and they will often share pictures and stories of their travels. I encourage them to share the emotions their memories evoke and recall the different sensations they remember, such as the smell of an orange grove in Spain or the feel of the sand on a beach in Hawaii. This activity is reflective of some of the approaches and techniques that will be discussed in more detail in the next section.

Theoretical Approaches and Techniques When Counseling Older Adults in a TMH Setting

There are many considerations when deciding which therapeutic approaches and interventions to utilize with older adult clients. One necessary consideration involves the cognitive level of the client. As adults grow older, there is often a decline in cognition, and TMH interventions must be adjusted as a result (Haron et al., 2016; Yang et al., 2009). Another consideration includes being aware of any medical conditions and mobility issues that are impacting the client. For example, clients who struggle with lung conditions may experience discomfort and distress when engaging in relaxed breathing exercises (Simms et al., 2011). In addition, clients with decreased visual or auditory abilities will need adjustments to the TMH platform so that they can receive ethical TMH services. In the next sections, we will explore a few of the approaches and techniques I have found to be the most helpful, including person-centered, mindfulness-based, and reminiscence therapy.

Person-Centered Therapy

As discussed earlier in the chapter, a person-centered approach helps to build rapport and develop a therapeutic alliance, as well as allow the client a safe space for self-expression (von Humboldt & Leal, 2012). As older adults transition into retirement age, they often face increased moments of ambiguity and uncertainty. A person-centered approach can provide security and encourage self-actualization to help the client cope with the uncertainty of the future and increase their sense of well-being (von Humboldt & Leal, 2012). The ability to convey genuine empathy, validation, unconditional positive regard, and nonjudgment becomes important as older adult clients address topics such as morality, grief, loss of independence and functional capacity, physical illness, and loneliness (von Humboldt & Leal, 2012; Wild et al., 2019).

In my clinical work with older adults, I have found that a person-centered approach becomes especially helpful when processing inherent topics of morality, grief, and loss. As adults age, they are confronted with declining personal health and functionality as well as the death of family and friends (Katherine et al., 2015; von Humboldt & Leal, 2012). The understanding that the life cycle is limited and nearing an end is also a common theme in sessions with the elderly (Kampfe, 2015; von Humboldt & Leal, 2012). Providing the client with a safe environment to express their emotions is extremely helpful in the grieving process (Kampfe, 2015). During this time, it is important to validate the client's emotions, whatever they may be, and avoid pushing outcomes (Kampfe, 2015; von Humboldt & Leal, 2012). In addition, it may be helpful for the client to identify and discuss the aspects of the loss and, in the case of the death of a family or friend, share their memories of and relationship with the person who died (Kampfe, 2015).

When thinking back on my TMH sessions that involved the processing of grief and loss, I remember working with a client who was having a difficult time after the death of his husband. As he processed his grief, he shared that their children and grandchildren were also struggling with the loss. I shared that it might be helpful for him and his family to create a scrapbook filled with memories of his husband outside of the session. He invited his children and grandchildren to create the memory book, and they worked on it over the next month. It included photographs, letters, and pictures the grandchildren had drawn of their favorite memories of their grandfather. During the sessions after the memory book was completed, I validated the client's emotions and listened with genuine empathy as he shared the book and his memories of his husband.

Mindfulness-Based Techniques

Older adult clients are likely to experience sleep disturbance, multiple stressors, depression, anxiety, and physical conditions that may cause muscle tension and general discomfort (Kampfe, 2015; Sun, 2021). Mindfulness-based techniques can aid older adult clients in coping with these concerns (Sun, 2021). These techniques might include relaxed breathing, progressive muscle relaxation, meditation, mindful walking, and guided imagery (Kampfe, 2015; Sun, 2021). As discussed earlier in the chapter, considerations must be made for the client's presenting medical conditions or impairments (Simms et al., 2011) so that the techniques meet the best needs of the client and do not cause harm.

One mindfulness-based activity that is easily adaptable to the TMH setting is a guided imagery visualization. There are many books and online resources that have prepared scripts that can be utilized with clients. It is important to first think about the intention for the guided imagery visualization. Is your client struggling with anxiety, depression, difficulty sleeping, chronic pain, and so forth? Choose a visualization that supports the treatment plan goals. Once you find a visualization that aligns with the treatment goal, you can lead your client through the visualization during a TMH session. After the visualization, you might ask your client some processing questions to gauge whether the practice was helpful and ask them to share what feelings came up for them. Following is an example of a brief guided imagery visualization and follow-up questions that I often use with older adults who are struggling with anxiety.

GUIDED IMAGERY SCRIPT EXAMPLE

Sit back and get comfortable in your chair. If you feel comfortable doing so, you can also close your eyes. We are going to do a little breathing to get centered. I'm going to have you breathe in for three counts and then breath out for three counts. Okay, breathe in 1 ... 2 ... 3 ... and breathe out 1 ... 2 ... 3. Again, breathe in 1 ... 2 ... 3 ... and breathe out 1 ... 2 ... 3. Now I want you to imagine you are in a relaxing place. Maybe it is in a garden full of your favorite flowers or on the beach during a sunny day, or maybe it is somewhere else. Get a clear picture of it in your mind. (Pause for about 5-10 seconds.) Now that you have a clear picture of the relaxing place, I want you to take a look around. What do you see? (Pause for 5-10 seconds.) What sounds can you hear? (Pause for 5-10 seconds.) Are there any smells in this place? (Pause for 5-10 seconds.) Do you feel anything beneath your feet or are your hands touching anything? (Pause for 5-10 seconds.) Is there anything that you can taste? (Pause for 5-10 seconds.) What emotions are you feeling in this place? (Pause for 5-10 seconds.) Take one last moment to experience your relaxing space. (Pause for 5-10 seconds.) Now start to wiggle your fingers and toes and slowly come back to the room. You can open your eyes when you are ready.

Reflective Questions

- How was that experience for you?
- Would you like to tell me about your relaxing place? (You can prompt with the five senses again if they are having trouble sharing.)
- What emotions did it bring up for you?
- Did you find the exercise helpful? (If not, ask them why they feel it was unhelpful.)

Reflective Activity

For my more artistically inclined clients who have access to art supplies in their home, I ask them to create a piece of art around their relaxing place. If they are unable to or do not feel like creating a piece of art, maybe they can find a postcard, photo, or clipping from a magazine that reminds them of their relaxing place. I discuss how it may be helpful for them to put the artwork, photo, or clipping somewhere where they will see it daily, such as the fridge or on their dresser. It can act as a reminder for them to use relaxation exercises throughout the day when they are feeling anxious.

Reminiscence Therapy

Reminiscence therapy is one of the most prominent interventions utilized with older adult clients and has been found to decrease depression (Hidayati, 2015; Soniya, 2015) and increase resilience, problem solving, quality of life, and self-esteem (Duru Aşiret & Dutkun, 2018; Melendez et al., 2015). Reminiscence therapy encourages older adults to become actively involved in sharing and reliving past events from their lives with the therapist (Soniya, 2015). The reminiscing experience may include sensory items such as music, photographs, and food to enhance the experience (Soniya, 2015). The reminiscing experience should be adjusted based on the cognitive level of the client. For example, the findings of a study by Haron et al. (2016) demonstrated that participants engaging in reminiscence therapy who presented with less cognitive decline appeared to do well with a formal and structured approach, while participants with higher cognitive decline appeared to do well with processes that used an informal and unstructured approach.

One example of a structured reminiscence therapy exercise I utilized with an older adult client during a TMH setting involved her love of art museums. This client had visited several famous art museums in the United States and Europe during her travels. I created a slideshow of work from one of the favorite museums she had visited, including some of the favorite artists she named. We looked at the slideshow together over the videoconferencing platform, and she shared the thoughts, emotions, and memories that surfaced as we looked at the artwork. She enjoyed the activity so much, she asked if I would create slideshows for a few other museums, and we viewed them during subsequent sessions. During this time, we had been working toward the goal of getting her motivated to engage in more of her hobbies to decrease her depressive symptoms. She reported that viewing the artwork inspired her to begin making art again during her free time. This in turn helped her to feel less lonely and increased her sense of well-being.

Upon reflecting on my years of working with older adults, I find myself thinking about the same characteristics I find helpful when working with adolescents: honesty, flexibility, humor, and creativity. I find that my older clients also echo my adolescent clients in expressing that the thing they find the most helpful about therapy is the presence of someone who validates their emotions and listens to them without judgment or condescension. They also often share that having weekly or biweekly therapy sessions helps them feel less alone in the world. As the chapter draws to a close, I want to impart a piece of advice I often find myself giving to new counselors: If you find yourself overthinking or getting lost in a session, tap into your foundational counseling skills and you will find your way back.

Chapter Summary

This chapter discussed specific considerations for providing TMH services to adolescents and older adults. TMH services help to provide therapy to adolescents and older adults who may have trouble accessing in-person services and allows them to receive services in their natural settings. While adolescents tend to be comfortable with utilizing technology, older adults may require assistance in adapting to the technology needed for TMH services.

It is important to note specific ethical considerations when counseling adolescent and older adult clients, including confidentiality, client rights and responsibilities when receiving care at a distance, age of majority, consent to care, client autonomy, beneficence, and mandated reporting. While it may seem overwhelming to think about these examples at first, keep in mind that you will have the support of your colleagues and supervisors as you move through learning how to address these considerations when you begin working with clients.

Developing a strong therapeutic alliance is the first step in building rapport and is associated with favorable and effective treatment outcomes. Building trust and reassuring clients that their privacy and confidentiality will be respected is of utmost importance. Often beginning sessions with adolescents and older adults involves the client and therapist getting to know each other through the sharing of important people, pets, items, and hobbies, as well as developing creative ways to engage the client, such as using music, videos, artwork, and photographs.

Creativity can also be applied when utilizing theoretical approaches and techniques to engage your client in a TMH setting. You learned about specific theoretical approaches and techniques, such as person-centered, cognitive behavioral therapy, psychoeducation, mindfulness-based, and reminiscence therapy. While each approach and technique has the ability to aid your client through the healing process, it is important to note that there is no substitute for the foundational skills of empathic listening, nonjudgment, genuineness, and validation.

APPLICATION ACTIVITY

Imagine you are working with an adolescent client in the beginning stages of counseling. Think about a creative rapport-building activity that you might suggest to a client. Find a partner/peer from your counseling program and meet on a video-enabled platform. Do a role-play of the creative activity with a classmate. Then reverse roles and engage in the role-play activity as if you are the client and your classmate is the therapist. After you have both had a turn being the counselor, reflect on the following prompts:

- What was it like to engage in the activity as a counselor?
- As the client, how did it feel to share about yourself?
- What constructive feedback do you have for your counselor on the experience?
- Do you think that the activity would be developmentally appropriate to utilize with the chosen population? Why or why not?

When you finish your discussion, switch the activity to consider working with an elderly client. Journal about your experience.

References

American Academy of Child and Adolescent Psychiatry Committee on Telepsychiatry & AACAP Committee on Quality Issues. (2017). Clinical update: Telepsychiatry with children and adolescents. *Journal of the American Academy of Child and Adolescent Psychiatry, 56*(10), 875–893. https://doi.org/10.1016/j.jaac.2017.07.008

American Bar Association Commission on Law and Aging, American Psychological Association, & National College of Probate Judges. (2006). *Judicial Determination of Capacity of Older Adults in Guardianship Proceedings.* https://www.apa.org/pi/aging/resources/guides/judges-diminished.pdf

American Counseling Association. (2014). *2014 ACA code of ethics.* https://www.counseling.org/docs/default-source/default-document-library/2014-code-of-ethics-finaladdress.pdf

American Psychological Association. (2017). *Guidelines for the practice of telepsychology.* https://www.apa.org/practice/guidelines/telepsychology

American Telemedicine Association. (2017, March). *Practice guidelines for telemental health with children and adolescents.* https://cdn2.hubspot.net/hubfs/5096139/NEW_ATA-Children-Adolescents-Guidelines-3.pdf

Batastini, A. B. (2016). Improving rehabilitative efforts for juvenile offenders through the use of telemental healthcare. *Journal of Child and Adolescent Psychopharmacology, 26*(3), 273–277. https://doi.org/10.1089/cap.2015.0011

Bearable LTD. (2022). *Bearable* (Version 1.0.360) [Mobile app]. https://bearable.app/

Boldy, D., Grenade, L., Lewin, G., Karol, E., & Burton, E. (2011). Older people's decisions regarding "ageing in place": A western Australian case study. *Australasian Journal on Ageing*, *30*(3), 136–142. https://doi.org/10.1111/j.1741-6612.2010.00469.x

Bronstein, L., Cook, K., & Lee, Y. (2021). Connecting grandparent caregivers through telemental health during COVID-19. *Innovation in Aging*, *5*(1), 262. https://doi.org/10.1093/geroni/igab046.1004

Bryant-Jefferies, R. (2017). *Counselling young people: Person-centered dialogues*. Taylor and Francis. https://doi.org/10.1201/9781315375489

Bush, S. S., Allen, R. S., & Molinari, V. A., III. (2017). *Ethical practice in geropsychology*. American Psychological Association. https://doi.org/10.1037/0000010-000

Chan, S. R., Torous, J., Hinton, L., & Yellowlees, P. (2014). Mobile tele-mental health: Increasing applications and a move to hybrid models of care. *Healthcare (Basel)*, *2*(2), 220–233. https://doi.org/10.3390/healthcare2020220

Chi, N. C., & Demiris, G. (2015). A systematic review of telehealth tools and interventions to support family caregivers. *Journal of Telemedicine and Telecare*, *21*(1), 37–44. https://doi.org/10.1177/1357633X14562734

Cirasola, A., Midgley, N., Fonagy, P., Consortium, I., & Martin, P. (2021). The therapeutic alliance in psychotherapy for adolescent depression: Differences between treatment types and change over time. *Journal of Psychotherapy Integration*, *32*(3), 326–341. https://doi.org/10.1037/int0000264

Comer, J. S., & Barlow, D. H. (2014). The occasional case against broad dissemination and implementation: Retaining a role for specialty care in the delivery of psychological treatments. *The American Psychologist*, *69*(1), 1–18. https://doi.org/10.1037/a0033582

Comer, J. S., & Myers, K. (2016). Future directions in the use of telemental health to improve the accessibility and quality of children's mental health services. *Journal of Child and Adolescent Psychopharmacology*, *26*(3), 296–300. https://doi.org/10.1089/cap.2015.0079

Duru Aşiret, G., & Dutkun, M. (2018). The effect of reminiscence therapy on the adaptation of elderly women to old age: A randomized clinical trial. *Complementary Therapies in Medicine*, *41*, 124–129. http://dx.doi.org/10.1016/j.ctim.2018.09.018

Egede, L. E., Frueh, C. B., Richardson, L. K., Acierno, R., Mauldin, P. D., Knapp, R. G., & Lejuez, C. (2009). Rationale and design: Telepsychology service delivery for depressed elderly veterans. *Trials*, *10*(1), 22–22. https://doi.org/10.1186/1745-6215-10-22

Forman, J. M., & McBride, R. G. (2010). Counselors' Role in Preventing Abuse of Older Adults: Clinical, Ethical, and Legal Considerations. *Adultspan Journal*, *9*(1), 4–13.

Gloff, N. E., LeNoue, S. R., Novins, D. K., & Myers, K. (2015). Telemental health for children and adolescents. *International Review of Psychiatry (Abingdon, England)*, *27*(6), 513–524. https://doi.org/10.3109/09540261.2015.1086322

Goldstein, F., & Glueck, D. (2016). Developing rapport and therapeutic alliance during telemental health sessions with children and adolescents. *Journal of Child and Adolescent Psychopharmacology*, *26*(3), 24–211. https://doi.org/10.1089/cap.2015.0022

Gümüs, F., Ergün, G., & Dikeç, G. (2020). Effect of psychoeducation on stress in parents of children with attention-deficit/hyperactivity disorder: A randomized controlled study. *Journal of Psychosocial Nursing and Mental Health Services, 58*(7), 1–41. https://doi.org/10.3928/02793695-20200506-01

Hage, E., Roo, J. P., van Offenbeek, Marjolein A. G., & Boonstra, A. (2013). Implementation factors and their effect on e-health service adoption in rural communities: A systematic literature review. *BMC Health Services Research, 13*(1), 19. https://doi.org/10.1186/1472-6963-13-19

Haron, H., Ali, M. C., & Sabri, S. M. (2016). Technology to support reminiscence therapy for elderly. *Information, 19*(10B), 4737. https://www.researchgate.net/publication/316279377_Technology_to_support_reminiscence_therapy_for_elderly

Heitzman-Powell, L. S., Buzhardt, J., Rusinko, L. C., & Miller, T. M. (2013). Formative evaluation of an ABA outreach training program for parents of children with autism in remote areas. *Focus Autism and Developmental Disabilities, 29*, 23–29.

Hidayati, L. N., Mustikasari, M., & Eka Putri, Y. S. (2015). Individual reminiscence therapy can decrease depression level on elderly at social homes. *Jurnal Ners (Surabaya), 10*(2), 222–232. https://doi.org/10.20473/jn.V10I22015.222-232

Himle, M. B., Freitag, M., Walther, M., Franklin, S. A., Ely, L., & Woods, D. W. (2012). A randomized pilot trial comparing videoconference versus face-to-face delivery of behavior therapy for childhood tic disorders. *Behaviour Research and Therapy, 50*(9), 565–570. https://doi.org/10.1016/j.brat.2012.05.009

Horvath, A. O. (2018). Research on the alliance: Knowledge in search of a theory. *Psychotherapy Research, 28*(4), 499–516. https://doi.org/10.1080/10503307.2017.1373204

Jones, A. M., Shealy, K. M., Reid-Quiñones, K., Moreland, A. D., Davidson, T. M., López, C. M., Barr, S. C., & de Arellano, M. A. (2014). Guidelines for establishing a telemental health program to provide evidence-based therapy for trauma-exposed children and families. *Psychological Services, 11*(4), 398–409. https://doi.org/10.1037/a0034963

Kampfe, C. M. (2015). *Counseling older people: Opportunities and challenges.* American Counseling Association.

Katherine, S. M., Ghesquiere, A., & Glickman, K. (2013). Bereavement and complicated grief. *Current Psychiatry Reports, 15*(11). http://doi.org/10.1007/s11920-013-0406-z

Kemp, J., Zhang, T., Inglis, F., Wiljer, D., Sockalingam, S., Crawford, A., Lo, B., Charow, R., Munnery, M., Singh Takhar, S., & Strudwick, G. (2020). Delivery of compassionate mental health care in a digital technology-driven age: Scoping review. *Journal of Medical Internet Research, 22*(3), e16263. https://doi.org/10.2196/16263

Kenny, R., Dooley, B., & Fitzgerald, A. (2015). Feasibility of "CopeSmart": A telemental health app for adolescents. *JMIR Mental Health, 2*(3), e22. https://doi.org/10.2196/mental.4370

Kroenke, K., Spitzer, R. L., & Williams, J. B. W. (2001). The PHQ-9. *Journal of General Internal Medicine: JGIM, 16*(9), 606–613. https://doi.org/10.1046/j.1525-1497.2001.016009606.x

Kroenke, K., Spitzer, R. L., Williams, J. B. W., & Lowe, B. (2006). A brief measure for assessing generalized anxiety disorder: The GAD-7. *Archives of Internal Medicine, 166*(10), 1092–1097. https://doi.org/10.1001/archinte.166.10.1092

Krysinska, K., Curtis, S., Lamblin, M., Stefanac, N., Gibson, K., Byrne, S., Thorn, P., Rice, S. M., McRoberts, A., Ferrey, A., Perry, Y., Lin, A., Hetrick, S., Hawton, K., & Robinson, J. (2020). Parents' experience and psychoeducation needs when supporting a young person who self-harms. *International Journal of Environmental Research and Public Health, 17*(10), 3662. https://doi.org/10.3390/ijerph17103662

Kuziemsky, C. E., Hunter, I., Gogia, S. B., Iyenger, S., Kulatunga, G., Rajput, V., Subbian, V., John, O., Kleber, A., Mandirola, H. F., Florez-Arango, J., Al-Shorbaji, N., Meher, S., Udayasankaran, J. G., & Basu, A. (2020). Ethics in telehealth: Comparison between guidelines and practice-based experience -the case for learning health systems. *Yearbook of Medical Informatics, 29*(1), 044–050. https://doi.org/10.1055/s-0040-1701976

Lau, N., Colt, S. F., Waldbaum, S., O'Daffer, A., Fladeboe, K., Yi-Frazier, J. P., McCauley, E., & Rosenberg, A. R. (2021). Telemental health for youth with chronic illnesses: Systematic review. *JMIR Mental Health, 8*(8), e30098–e30098. https://doi.org/10.2196/30098

Melendez, J. C., Fortuna, F. B., Sales, A., & Mayordomo, T. (2015). Effect of integrative reminiscence therapy on depression, well-being, integrity, self-esteem, and life satisfaction in older adults. *The Journal of Positive Psychology, 10*(3), 240–247.

Myers, K., Vander Stoep, A., Zhou, C., McCarty, C. A., & Katon, W. (2015). Effectiveness of a telehealth service delivery model for treating attention deficit/hyperactivity disorder: A community-based randomized controlled trial. *Journal of the American Academy of Child and Adolescent Psychiatry, 54*(4), 263–274. https://doi.org/10.1016/j.jaac.2015.01.009

National Adult Protective Services Association. (2018). *NAPSA Adult Protective Services Abuse Registry National Report.* https://www.napsa-now.org/wp-content/uploads/2022/04/APS-Abuse-Registry-Report-2.pdf

Nelson, E., Barnard, M., & Cain, S. (2006). Feasibility of telemedicine intervention for childhood depression. *Counselling and Psychotherapy Research, 6*(3), 191–195. https://doi.org/10.1080/14733140600862303

Nelson, E., & Bui, T. (2010). Rural telepsychology services for children and adolescents. *Journal of Clinical Psychology, 66*(4), 490–501. https://doi.org/10.1002/jclp.20682

Nelson, E., & Patton, S. (2016). Using videoconferencing to deliver individual therapy and pediatric psychology interventions with children and adolescents. *Journal of Child and Adolescent Psychopharmacology, 26*(3), 212–220. https://doi.org/10.1089/cap.2015.0021

Oshima, F., William, M., Takahashi, N., Tsuchiyagaito, A., Kuwabara, H., Shiina, A., Seto, M., Hongo, M., Iwama, Y., Hirano, Y., Sutoh, C., Taguchi, K., Yoshida, T., Kawasaki, Y., Ozawa, Y., Masuya, J., Sato, N., Nakamura, S., Kuno, M., . . . & Shimizu, E. (2020). Cognitive-behavioral family therapy as psychoeducation for adolescents with high-functioning autism spectrum disorders: Aware and care for my autistic traits (ACAT) program study protocol for a pragmatic multisite randomized controlled trial. *Trials, 21*(1), 814. https://doi.org/10.1186/s13063-020-04750-z

Peek, S. T. M., Luijkx, K. G., Vrijhoef, H. J. M., Nieboer, M. E., Aarts, S., van der Voort, C. S., Rijnaard, M. D., & Wouters, E. J. M. (2019). Understanding changes and stability in the long-term use of technologies by seniors who are aging in place: A dynamical framework. *BMC Geriatrics, 19*(1), 236–236. https://doi.org/10.1186/s12877-019-1241-9

Pew Research Center. (2021). *Mobile Technology and Home Broadband.* https://www.pewresearch.org/internet/2021/06/03/mobile-technology-and-home-broadband-2021/

Pruitt, L. D., Luxton, D. D., & Shore, P. (2014). Additional clinical benefits of home-based tele-mental health treatments. *Professional Psychology, Research and Practice, 45*(5), 340–346. https://doi.org/10.1037/a0035461

Reese, R., Jamison, R., Wendland, M., Fleming, K., Braun, M., Schuttler, J., & Turek, J. (2013). Evaluating interactive videoconferencing for assessing symptoms of autism. *Telemedicine and e-Health, 19*(9), 671–677. https://doi.org/10.1089/tmj.2012.0312

Reyes-Portillo, J. A., Mufson, L., Greenhill, L. L., Gould, M. S., Fisher, P. W., Tarlow, N., & Rynn, M. A. (2014). Web-based interventions for youth internalizing problems: A systematic review. *Journal of the American Academy of Child and Adolescent Psychiatry, 53*(12), 1254–1270.e5. https://doi.org/10.1016/j.jaac.2014.09.005

Roble Ridge Software LLC. (2022). *Moodfit* (Version 2.27) [Mobile app]. https://www.getmoodfit.com/

Shang, Z., Arnaert, A., Hindle, Y., Debe, Z., Côté-Leblanc, G., & Saadi, A. (2020). Experiences of telemental health providers and support staff serving Indigenous patients of northern Canada. *Research Square.* https://doi.org/10.21203/rs.3.rs-36224/v1

Simms, D. C., Gibson, K., & O'Donnell, S. (2011). To use or not to use: Clinicians' perceptions of telemental health. *Canadian Psychology = Psychologie Canadienne, 52*(1), 41–51. https://doi.org/10.1037/a0022275

Soniya, G. (2015). Reminiscence therapy to reduce depression among elderly. *International Journal of Nursing Education, 7*(2), 160–164. https://doi.org/10.5958/0974-9357.2015.00095.1

Spence, S. H., Holmes, J. M., March, S., & Lipp, O. V. (2006). The feasibility and outcome of clinic plus internet delivery of cognitive-behavior therapy for childhood anxiety. *Journal of Consulting and Clinical Psychology, 74*(3), 614–621. https://doi.org/10.1037/0022-006X.74.3.614

Stephan, S., Lever, N., Bernstein, L., Edwards, S., & Pruitt, D. (2016). Telemental health in schools. *Journal of Child and Adolescent Psychopharmacology, 26*(3), 266–272. https://doi.org/10.1089/cap.2015.0019

Storch, E. A., Caporino, N. E., Morgan, J. R., Lewin, A. B., Rojas, A., Brauer, L., Larson, M. J., & Murphy, T. K. (2011). Preliminary investigation of web-camera delivered cognitive-behavioral therapy for youth with obsessive-compulsive disorder. *Psychiatry Research, 189*(3), 407–412. https://doi.org/10.1016/j.psychres.2011.05.047

Sun, X., Xie, L., Feng, X., Xia, X., He, Y., Tan, L., & Zhao, H. (2021). Evaluation of the application effect of online mindfulness-based cognitive therapy in the health management of elderly patients with COPD during the novel coronavirus pneumonia epidemic. *Journal of Evidence-Based Psychotherapies, 21*(1), 57–67. https://doi.org/10.24193/jebp.2021.1.4

Tillfors, M., Andersson, G., Ekselius, L., Furmark, T., Lewenhaupt, S., Karlsson, A., & Carlbring, P. (2011). A randomized trial of internet-delivered treatment for social anxiety disorder in high school students. *Cognitive Behaviour Therapy, 40*(2), 147–157. https://doi.org/10.1080/16506073.2011.555486

University of Michigan. (2013). *Psychoeducation: Trauma.* https://trailstowellness.org/materials/cbt-and-mindfulness-groups/resources/psychoeducation-trauma

Vander Stoep, A., McCarty, C. A., Zhou, C., Rockhill, C. M., Schoenfelder, E. N., & Myers, K. (2017). The children's attention-deficit hyperactivity disorder telemental health treatment study:

Caregiver outcomes. *Journal of Abnormal Child Psychology, 45*(1), 27–43. https://doi.org/10.1007/s10802-016-0155-7

von Humboldt, S., & Leal, I. (2012). Building bridges: Person-centered therapy with older adults. *European Journal of Business and Social Sciences, 1*(8), 23–32. https://www.researchgate.net/publication/319315622_Building_bridges_Person-centered_therapy_with_older_adults

Wang, J., Du, Y., Coleman, D., Peck, M., Myneni, S., Kang, H., & Gong, Y. (2019). Mobile and connected health technology needs for older adults aging in place: Cross-sectional survey study. *JMIR Aging, 2*(1), e13864. https://doi.org/10.2196/13864

Wild, B., Heider, D., Schellberg, D., Böhlen, F., Schöttker, B., Muhlack, D. C., König, H., & Slaets, J. (2019). Caring for the elderly: A person-centered segmentation approach for exploring the association between health care needs, mental health care use, and costs in Germany. *PLoS One, 14*(12). http://dx.doi.org/10.1371/journal.pone.0226510

Xie, Y. J., Dixon, F., Yee, O. M., Zhang, J. Y., Chen, A., DeAngelo, S., Yellowlees, P., Hendren, R., & Schweitzer, J. B. (2013, March 12). A study on the effectiveness of videoconferencing on teaching parent training skills to parents of children with ADHD. Telemedicine and e-Health, 192–199. http://doi.org/10.1089/tmj.2012.0108

Yang, J. A., Garis, J., Jackson, C., & McClure, R. (2009). Providing psychotherapy to older adults in home: Benefits, challenges, and decision-making guidelines. *Clinical Gerontologist, 32*(4), 333–346. https://doi.org/10.1080/07317110902896356

Credits

CHAPTER 9

Application of Telemental Health, Part 3

Couples, Families, and Groups

Nicole M. Arcuri Sanders and Alisha Davis

Alone we can do so little; together we can do so much.

–Helen Keller

Learning Objectives

After reading this chapter, you should be able to do the following:

1. Identify unique attributes of telemental health services for couples, families, and groups
2. Recognize ethical implications related to telemental health services for couples, families, and groups
3. Critically examine the learned information with case applications for telemental health work with couples, families, and groups

Introduction

By this point in the text, you have read and reflected on a lot of information relevant to the practice of telemental health counseling and may be wondering, "What have I signed up for?" Please know that this information is not intended to intimidate you, but is instead intended to share information in great detail to support your confidence in feeling competent. We say this because you may be feeling overwhelmed in considering all the various aspects that come with not only the virtual platforms (e.g., legal and ethical implications) but also with providing counseling services to an individual client

Image 9.1

from a distance. This chapter will ask you to apply your skills to meet the needs of multiple clients at once. Telemental health counseling services offered to couples, families, and groups require counselors to exercise particular considerations prior to commencing, throughout, and with aftercare of services.

When bringing more than one client into the session, each client's well-being needs to be accounted for (American Counseling Association [ACA], 2014, A.1.a). This requires the counselor to ensure they conduct thorough intakes of all of the clients, whether they are seeking couple, family, or group counseling services. Each client is unique and deserves to feel heard and validated regardless of the setting in which they seek counseling services. Thus, just as with in-person counseling, the counselor needs to build and maintain therapeutic rapport with each client throughout the counseling process. Informed consent must be received by each client prior to commencing services (ACA, 2014, B.4). With couples, family, and group work comes variances in the informed consent process. Additionally, ethical and legal implications need to be considered for work with each client and with the system as a whole (e.g., couple, family, or group). These implications will be elaborated on later in this chapter in accordance with each system.

This task may seem daunting, but I encourage you to reflect back on your journey thus far and realize just how capable you are. Adding additional clients to the case does take additional deliberation; however, the task is not impossible. Others have done it, and so can you! This chapter intends to break down work with couples, families, and groups via telemental health with examples to highlight implementation as well as ethical and legal implications. At the end of this chapter, you will be invited to reflect on the information shared and create a plan to support you in your efforts of working with couples, families, and groups in a virtual platform. To start off, we will review legal and ethical implications needed for couples, family, and group work as well as unique virtual platform elements to consider.

Legal and Ethical Guidance When Working With Couples, Families, or Groups

First and foremost, prior to providing any counseling services to couples, families, and/or groups, you will need to ensure the parameters of your state law. For instance, some states may require additional coursework or experience, which may result in a specialty designation on your license to be permitted to conduct such services (e.g., California for couples and families at the time of this writing). The type of services may also be limited to the particular license held. For instance, in some states, licensed counselors have permission to provide individual and group counseling; however, only licensed marriage and family counselors can conduct couple and/or family sessions. Therefore, prior to even debating about extending your services to include couples, families, and groups, it is necessary to consult your state licensing board.

If your state legally defines your scope of practice to include family, couple, and/or group work, you are now ready to explore what ethical responsibilities you have. It's time to pull out your handy American Counseling Association (ACA) and/or American Mental Health Counseling Association (AMHCA) code of ethics again. First, you need to examine an important question for yourself: Do you possess the training, knowledge, and confidence to provide such services effectively to clients (i.e., competence; ACA, 2014, C.2; AMHCA, 2020, C.1)?

If you feel ill-equipped, it will be your ethical obligation to seek professional development (ACA, 2014, C.2.f; AMHCA, 2020, C.1.f, n) prior to offering the services. Once you feel confident and competent, you will need to ensure you have an informed consent that can clearly denote everything required to conduct telehealth services (e.g., state law and ethical codes) just as you did with individual clients, but also to include any specific variances applicable to couples, families, and groups. In Chapter 2, you explored ACA codes specific to telemental health counseling. In the following box, we highlight some additional ACA codes that are particularly relevant to couples, family, and group work.

TABLE 9.1   ACA Ethical Codes Relevant to Couples, Family, and Group Work

ACA (2014) Ethical Codes	Counselor Considerations
A.2.c. Developmental and Cultural Sensitivity Counselors communicate information in ways that are both developmentally and culturally appropriate.	All members of the counseling process (couple, family, and/or group services) should have the opportunity to feel validated and understood. To establish a therapeutic relationship with each client, the counselor will need to adjust their communication practices to support understanding of all their clients, even young children involved.

(Continued)

ACA (2014) Ethical Codes	Counselor Considerations
A.8. Multiple Clients When a counselor agrees to provide counseling services to two or more persons who have a relationship, the counselor clarifies at the outset which person or persons are clients and the nature of the relationships the counselor will have with each involved person. If it becomes apparent that the counselor may be called on to perform potentially conflicting roles, the counselor will clarify, adjust, or withdraw from roles appropriately. **B.4.b. Couples and Family Counseling** In couples and family counseling, counselors clearly define who is considered "the client" and discuss expectations and limitations of confidentiality. Counselors seek agreement and document in writing such agreement among all involved parties regarding the confidentiality of information. In the absence of an agreement to the contrary, the couple or family is considered the client.	When working with a couple or family, it is necessary to establish the identified client(s). You will need to address how this will impact your work with them together in session and what your role will look like. It will be important for the client(s) to understand that their well-being is a priority for you. Including this information in the informed consent is helpful, as the informed consent is a living document that can be adjusted if changes occur during the process (e.g., role changes/members withdraw, etc.).
A.9.a. Screening Counselors screen prospective group counseling/therapy participants. To the extent possible, counselors select members whose needs and goals are compatible with the goals of the group, who will not impede the group process, and whose well-being will not be jeopardized by the group experience.	The well-being of all your clients in the group needs to be considered. In order to foster therapeutic progress for all members within a group, potential clients need to be screened for fit. Despite having the same diagnosis, experience, and/or concerns, some group dynamics will not support therapeutic growth for clients.
A.9.b. Protecting Clients In a group setting, counselors take reasonable precautions to protect clients from physical, emotional, or psychological trauma.	In addition to proactively screening (A.9.a), it is also important to establish, within the informed consent, the risks and benefits involved with participation (e.g., exploring difficult topics that have intense emotional responses). It is also important to plan for additional resources that can be utilized within sessions and to support aftercare follow-up.
B.4.a. Group Work In group work, counselors clearly explain the importance and parameters of confidentiality for the specific group.	Counselors have the ethical and legal obligation to maintain client confidentiality (outside of established exceptions). With group members, they are encouraged to maintain confidentiality; however, there is not a guarantee that they will do so.

ACA (2014) Ethical Codes	Counselor Considerations
B.6.e. Client Access Counselors provide reasonable access to records and copies of records when requested by competent clients. Counselors limit the access of clients to their records, or portions of their records, only when there is compelling evidence that such access would cause harm to the client. Counselors document the request of clients and the rationale for withholding some or all of the records in the files of clients. In situations involving multiple clients, counselors provide individual clients with only those parts of records that relate directly to them and do not include confidential information related to any other client.	Client access to records needs to be included and discussed as part of the informed consent. Members need to be aware of who has access to clinical records. If one client from the system requests documentation of their progress, the counselor will need to remind them of what was agreed on within the informed consent process.

Couple, Family, and Group Virtual Platform Elements

There are numerous unique considerations for family, couple, and group telemental health counseling that extend beyond the facets needed for individual telemental health sessions. Your clients may have varied levels of confidence and competence with technology as well as developmental and cognitive capability implications. Furthermore, you can have clients in more than one location, which requires additional considerations with choice of platform since some services can only support the counselor and one client location. Other services allow for more people to access at once from multiple locations; however, they may charge different amounts for HIPAA-compliant platforms. As such, it is important to be aware of how many clients will need to access the virtual space during the same time. You will then need to ensure you select a platform that can support this number while also considering the compliance factors associated with HIPAA. At the start of the COVID-19 pandemic, many counselors who offered group counseling services were left struggling to find platforms that were HIPAA compliant and allowed for more than two or a few participants. The urgency brought about during the pandemic for many counselors has taught us a valuable lesson in being prepared for the unexpected. As such, I strongly encourage you to have a plan in place, even if you believe you will work with groups in face-to-face settings. It will be better for all counselors to be prepared to shift if and when it is needed so that you can provide your clients with continuity of care (ACA, 2014, A.12).

Once you establish the HIPAA-compliant platform that will meet the needs of your counseling service, a good question to ask is "What will the setup look like in terms of where the clients will be during the session?" For instance, should a couple be in the same room sharing the same camera space, or should each client have their own camera view and commence the sessions from a place they feel most comfortable? Can this fluctuate throughout the sessions? Will this vary for different couples, families, and groups? Is it okay for some family or group members to share a camera while others have their own? What if it is a parent helping a child/teen and they attend together in one camera lens? Could this cause other family members to believe there is an alliance stronger with some more than others? Could the perception of camera placement exasperate concerns presented by clients? There are so many questions here to consider and answers the counselor needs to guide clients with parameters from the start of the counseling experience. These parameters need a clear purpose, and if changed throughout the duration of services, need to be discussed. Counselors should be prepared to substantiate their reasoning as clients can wonder how the parameters in place may support their experience in counseling. This is where you get to put your master's-level writing skills into effect with your informed consent (also known as a *professional disclosure statement*) and make sure you substantiate your design to support best practices for your clients (ACA, 2014, C.7.a). Reviewing relevant research on family systems and structural implications to units (e.g., Bowen, structural, and strategic theory) can also be helpful as you consider client placement in virtual settings.

Let's practice! Here are a few examples of client dynamics you may want to prepare to address:

- Mom and Dad are in the same house and use the same computer. Their teenage son is on his phone in his room in the parent's house, and their daughter is at college in her dorm room 3 hours away in a different state.
- Husband and wife are seeking couple's counseling due to lack of intimacy concerns. Husband attends from a hotel room as he travels for work. Wife attends from their home, usually in their bedroom with their two children (ages 4 and 9) sleeping down the hall.
- There are seven group members. Each member has a diagnosis of generalized anxiety disorder. Each client uses a headset (e.g., headphones or AirPods). Four of the group members attend from a private space in their home. Two members attend from their kitchen; one of these members lives alone and has no other person in the home during this time; the other lives with a roommate who sometimes is seen in the background grabbing something out of the fridge. One member attends from the porch in their backyard.

VOICES FROM THE FIELD

Have you noticed anything different in your clients between practicing in a telemental health setting versus face-to-face?

"Clients show a different side of themselves on video telehealth—they are much more vulnerable and do not put on a show. [T]hey are more real—I see them in their cars, in their homes, at their workplaces ... . It helps me get a broader picture of their world."

—Melissa Lee-Tammeus, PhD, LMHC, Jacksonville, FL

Take a few minutes to reflect on the following prompts with regard to each of these scenarios:

- Is the clients' freedom to share limited by location?
- Is it possible an authoritative power is gaining more power by sharing one screen and not having a separate space?
- What other potential concerns may be present?

Before we get started applying ethical, legal, and platform implications to actual possible scenarios, we encourage you to engage in this next exercise to gain a better mind-set that you will need to support working with multiple clients at once.

- Please join three to five classmates, friends, and/or family members in a virtual space (e.g., Zoom, GoogleMeet) for anywhere between 30 and 60 minutes. Remember an average counseling session ranges from 50–60 minutes. Remember this is not a counseling session as you are in training, but rather this is an opportunity to practice and reflect on facilitating communication with multiple people in a virtual space.
- Ask the general question to get the conversation started, "How is everyone?"

  - Pay attention to who speaks first, who may not join in, and who may be distracted versus who is fully engaged. Who needs to be prompted to join the conversation versus who needs to be asked to give someone else a chance to share? Take inventory of both nonverbal and verbal behaviors that support your understanding of their involvement in the group.

- Depending on your group, if you need an additional topic to keep the conversation flowing, consider what connects you all and ask about this using an open-ended question. This is similar to the presenting concern that brings clients for counseling services.

- - Once again, take inventory of both nonverbal and verbal behaviors that support your understanding of the members' involvement in the group.
  - If the conversation comes to a stagnant point, utilize your foundational counseling skills to support deeper conversation (e.g., open-ended questions, reflecting, paraphrasing).

- At approximately 5–10 minutes, before ending your time together, summarize the session and invite anyone else who would like to add something prior to wrapping up your time together.

  - - Once again, take inventory of both nonverbal and verbal behaviors that support your understanding of the members' involvement in the group.

- Bring closure to your group and ensure all members disconnect.

After this experience, notate what this experience was like for you in the facilitator role. Reflect on any aspects that appeared to come naturally as well as others that seemed more daunting or difficult. Consider this experience as you are introduced to the following cases so that you can understand how you may navigate working with the couple, family, and/or group with their presenting concern while being mindful of the virtual space the session is being conducted in.

Couple, Family, and Group Case Applications for Telemental Health Practice

This next sections are intended to provide counselors-in-training with examples of how counselors are currently navigating the dynamics related to working with couples, families, and groups using telemental health platforms. As a reminder, the various ethical and legal implications noted in the previous sections need to be considered. However, this next section will focus more on providing an understanding of how to maneuver in real-time with the clients using distance technologies in virtual counseling settings.

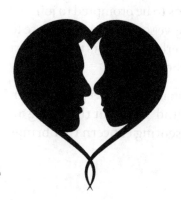

Couples

Couple's counseling is a unique therapeutic modality. Working within the dynamic of two individuals whose relationship may very well be on the precipice of termination can prove to be both challenging and immensely rewarding. Assisting couples in translating their thoughts and feelings and clarifying the desired path forward requires a secure grasp of foundational counseling skills, firm boundaries, and balance.

Image 9.2

Couples will seek counseling at various stages in their relationships. Research has shown that poor relationship health can contribute to elevated symptoms of anxiety and depression and signal an increased chance of relationship termination (Duncan et al., 2020). We know that women are more likely to initiate requests for counseling and that couples tend to wait to seek treatment longer than individuals (Parnell et al., 2018). When working with couples, counselors need to be culturally competent and adjust interventions to remove any bias and seek additional training when needed (Scott et al., 2019).

The benefits of telemental health for couples are substantial. Clients can be seen in the comfort of their homes, thereby removing barriers to accessing care. Couples may experience conflicting schedules, transportation limitations, or experience compounding mental health symptoms, which may prohibit traveling to an office for appointments (Wrape & McGinn, 2019). Telemental health also provides the opportunity for couples who may travel for work or are in long-distance relationships to obtain services (Hertlein et al., 2021; Wrape & McGinn, 2019).

Virtual couples counseling is not without special considerations. Two essential factors for telemental health are confidentiality and safety (Wrape & McGinn, 2019). One in three women and one in four men experience intimate partner violence (IPV) in their lifetimes (NCADV, 2021), and the rates of IPV for the LGBTQ community are disproportionately higher than the national average (Whitfield et al., 2021). Being prepared to address these facets unique to telemental health with couples can improve efficacy and ensure appropriate therapeutic boundaries and the clients' safety (Hertlein et al., 2021).

The next section will provide you with a couple's case examining various ethical implications addressed in previous sections while accounting for the telehealth format.

Case Application: A Couple Living Apart

For this next section, please review these helpful tips to support you in navigating telemental health couple work.

- Prior to commencing counseling sessions:
  - Check state laws pertaining to telemental health services with clients residing in the state as well as outside of the state and/or traveling out of their state of residence. It is important to be mindful that commencing counseling services extends to the location of the client and counselor during the time of the services.
  - Identify who is the client. According to ACA (2014) codes of ethics, the client needs to be clearly defined and agreed on by the couple in writing or all are considered the client (e.g., couple; B.4.b). Furthermore, each individual involved, whether established to be the client or not, is required to agree, in writing, to understanding limits to confidentiality when receiving couple's counseling services.

- With informed consent, ensure to have the address of the residence of the clients. Locate emergency and referral services prior to beginning sessions for the clients.
- Clients should be requested to provide you with information concerning out-of-state travel if they want to continue their telemental health services with you during that time so that the counselor can in advance check with state laws to ensure they can continue to provide services to the client during that time (e.g., work trip, vacation).
- Obtain a signed release of information form for the duration of counseling services with the counselor for the counselor to contact the local emergency service provider.
- Confirm time zones due to variance in state locations.

- During counseling session:

  - Particularly when using a telemental health platform outside of video (e.g., chat), confirm the identity of your client. Also, at the start of each session, ask clients to confirm their specific location (e.g., address) and phone number in case the internet connection is disrupted and/or a crisis situation presents. If different from the area indicated with informed consent, identify local emergency service information prior to commencing the session.

Husband (Xavier) and Wife (Jennifer) have been married for 16 months and dated 3 years prior to marriage. Two months ago, Jennifer was diagnosed with postpartum depression 2 months after their first child was born (child is 6 months old). Jennifer reported a lack of intimacy in their relationship after the birth of their child. Xavier indicated that he recently had a one-night stand with another woman 2 months ago, and he blames his decision at the time on the fact that his wife "only has time for the baby now" and does not want to be intimate.

Xavier is in the military and recently relocated (1 week ago) without his family (wife and 6-month-old child). The couple shared with Tyron (counselor) that Jennifer's family lives locally to where she currently lives, so she wanted to stay for support and help with their child since Xavier is expected to deploy within the next year. Xavier shared that he also believes Jennifer decided to stay because he was unfaithful 2 months ago. Jennifer admits that she does not attend any more military installation activities because she feels embarrassed by what her husband has done and feels like everyone else knows as well.

Prior to engaging in couple's counseling, both Xavier and Jennifer completed an intake/biopsychosocial assessment and submitted this along with their signed informed consent, which included their personalized code words to identify themselves during sessions via encrypted email to Tyron. It was established that both Jennifer and Xavier will be considered the client. Tyron confirmed he could provide services via telemental health for both clients' locations as he is licensed in both states.

At the start of the first session, Tyron introduced himself and welcomed Xavier and Jennifer. He then immediately asked them to identify themselves by typing their individually established code words from their informed consent (*client verification*). After each client's identity was verified with their code word, Tyron gave them an opportunity to ask any questions concerning the informed consent. Tyron reviewed limitations of confidentiality and sought verbal consent to commence couples counseling.

From there, Tyron immediately asked both Xavier and Jennifer to respond to his private chat with their current location (e.g., address) and phone number where they can be reached in the event they get disconnected or if needed for emergency purposes (*legal implication*). The counselor reviewed the purpose of understanding their location for client's safety considerations, as noted in the informed consent they both just agreed to. After Tyron received the information, he thanked them and reminded them this will happen at the start of each session.

As Tyron proceeds with the session, he is mindful of both clients, their locations, and the aspect that despite being married, they are currently at separate residences. One client is seeking possible marital resolution, while another is considering dissolving the marriage. He is supportive of both clients in navigating their perspectives while also considering the background of their lives in their real-time space. What we mean by this is that Xavier is located in an apartment unfamiliar to Jennifer while Jennifer is in what was previously considered their home with their daughter. Jennifer also has family in the home assisting with their daughter when she has these sessions. Confidentiality of both clients needs to be considered while addressing their feelings about their personal as well as each other's settings. Jennifer may feel disconnected from where Xavier now calls home while Xavier may feel cut off from what he once referred to as his home. Understanding the feelings of the clients in their space is important in supporting the clients in being vulnerable.

Counseling Families

Family systems counseling provides the unique opportunity to identify the strengths of a family unit and areas where communication breakdowns and destructive behavioral patterns may be playing out. Addressing these areas of concern can provide bright prospects for repairing disconnect and healing relationships between family members. Counselors must be prepared

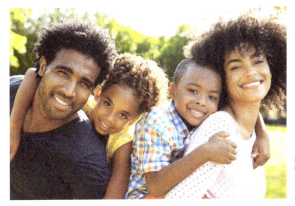

Image 9.3

to receive and interpret a vast amount of information—instead of one or two clients, you now may have four or five!

Family units come in various shapes and sizes, and it is not uncommon for even close-knit families to be separated geographically. Imagine trying to coordinate a scheduled visit with a set of parents, stepparents, and a teenager! Telemental health provides the platform to connect struggling families with a counselor who can assist them in building a path forward. Establishing clear and concise communication, ground rules, and procedures for virtual family sessions is a must. The counselor will need to attend to each member, be prepared to utilize a range of skills to maintain harmony and address technical issues as they arise (Herlein et al., 2020). It is critical that each client feels heard and validated. It is important for counselors to proactively set guidance, boundaries, and plans to promote healthy and effective communication and to support clients understanding their story and conveying that their well-being is of utmost priority.

Research has shown virtual family counseling to be effective and well received by clients (Tuckson et al., 2017; Wrape & McGinn, 2019). Special considerations for utilizing telemental health with families include confidentiality, safety, attending to several clients, building therapeutic rapport within the family, and coordination and implementation of treatment planning (Blumer et al., 2015; Wrape & McGinn, 2019). These factors will be further highlighted through the clients' scenario.

Case Application: A Family Separating

For this next section, let's build on the tips presented in the couple's section with these additional points to support you in navigating telemental health family work:

- Counselors clearly establish ground rules so that all members of the family understand the expectation that all will have opportunities to share without unnecessary interruption.
- Counselors need to be aware of the numerous member nonverbals that often occur simultaneously (screen clarity is helpful here, which requires a strong and stable internet connection).
- Counselors are mindful of possible authority dynamics that may interfere with the counseling process for the family. For instance, if parents were on one camera and highlighted in one box, and children separately in other boxes, this could reinforce an us-versus-them dynamic within the system. When warranted, a strategy that may be considered is to ask each client in a video session to log in from their own device so that groupings do not occur.

For this hypothetical case, the family is experiencing paramount adjustments as a whole as well as for numerous individuals within the family. They have reached out to Shandra, a counselor offering family sessions in her practice. The family consists of Dad (42; Michael), Mom (41; Nicole), and three children (8 [Sam], 16 [John], and

19 [Tiffany]). Michael retired from the Navy 3 months ago after 22 years of service. Michael wants to find a part-time job for extra spending money and to stay busy but does not want to initiate a new career. Nicole has been a stay-at-home mother for the past 19 years but now wants to go back to college and finish her degree in education while working part-time in the schools to develop a network. Nicole stresses this is a great time for her to do this since Michael can be home to attend to the children's needs more.

Prior to the family session, Shandra met with family members via individual video sessions to complete an intake. Shandra found this a good opportunity to understand each of the members of the family separately to gain more insight concerning the family dynamic and clients' perceptions of the family.

During the third session, after verifying each client's identity with their code word, obtaining current client locations, and performing initial check-ins with each family member, Michael (bottom left square of the telemental health platform) asked if he can share something first. Michael, now 4 months retired, says, "I don't know how to say this, so I am just going to say it. I know you all seem to really like Virginia, but I cannot stand it. I do not know how everyone doesn't seem to mind the traffic and living on top of each other. I just need more space, and this area does not offer it. I talked to your mom, and she has agreed that I can share this with you because she has shared that I seem angry at home and that you kids should know that it is not you I am angry at. I don't want to leave you all, but I think I need to step away." (See table visualize how each client and the counselor were displayed on the telemental health platform.)

Tiffany (19-year-old daughter)	Sam (8-year-old son)	John (16-year-old son)
Michael (Dad)	Shandra (Counselor)	Nicole (Mom)

The telemental health platform squares all began to highlight as each client camera and mic activated. In the far top-left corner of the screen, Shandra heard Tiffany laugh and observed her roll her eyes. Sam, top center square, started to cry, and John's face (right-top square) began to redden. Nicole (bottom-right square) put her head down and broke eye contact with everyone as Michael spoke.

The nonverbals here were extremely important to the content of the session and needed to be addressed for all by Shandra. Additionally, the counselor needed to remind the family members (clients) of the ground rules for their sessions. Shandra acknowledged the various reactions, both verbal and nonverbal, she witnessed with Michael's share. She reminded them that being honest and vulnerable can be difficult for anyone, and that as a family it had been previously decided to support honest and open communication and the right for all to finish their share without being interrupted even if another member of the family did not agree. Shandra then asked Michael if he would be willing to finish sharing. Michael, with his eyes closed, took a deep breath and then said, "I think I need to step away and go to the family ranch out in Texas."

Shandra thanked Michael for honestly sharing and noted how she recognized again the different reactions in the room from the family members. Shandra invited everyone to process what they just heard. Prior to getting started, Shandra reminded the family members that all of their thoughts deserve to be shared in a space without interruption by others. Tiffany immediately said, "Why bother? He does whatever he wants anyway." And then chaos appeared to erupt with the family members talking over one another as they shared their thoughts about what Michael said.

> "That's not true, I do everything for my family." (Michael)
>
> "You don't have the military as an excuse anymore. You don't want to be here, so just leave. There are no more ships or trainings that you are needed at. You finally get time with your family now and you still don't want to be here." (Tiffany)
>
> [Heavy breathing] (Michael)
>
> [Gasps] (John and Sam)
>
> [Both hands covering her face and crying] (Nicole)

Shandra interjected to provide both support to the family and order to the session. "It is evident that there is a great deal of emotion concerning this topic. I want to hear you all and understand your feelings, but I cannot do this when everyone is talking at the same time. Also, this is not fair for each of you because you are not getting the respect you have all indicated you believe your family should offer each other. Please remember the guidelines we have in place to demonstrate respect for one another even if what is shared results in strong emotions. Please know that you will have the opportunity to share when you have the floor." The family members then resumed their sharing, following the guidelines for respectful communication.

A lot happened during this session. Using a telemental health platform proved beneficial as it allowed all members to be part of the session in an equal manner (e.g., not just college child joining in from a virtual platform as everyone else was in the same room). However, the distance platform also presented some challenges. For instance, when clients are in a space that is familiar to them, it may also support behaviors that they may not demonstrate in more public settings like at a counseling center. Therefore, having clear parameters is needed to support a therapeutic session for all members. Additionally, nonverbals had to be addressed for clarity at times. Due to client access to space and technology, often counselors are limited to seeing their upper body only. Therefore, the counselor has to be in tune to these nonverbals and address this limitation when needed to check in and raise awareness. A stable internet connection is also important to ensure the counselor can receive a clear picture of the clients throughout the entirety of the session.

Groups

So you want to conduct counseling groups online? Great! There are a few considerations before you start your journey. Virtual group work can be exciting, challenging, and very rewarding. Group roles and dynamics are fascinating! As with all group work, the facilitator will need strong basic counseling skills and be well versed in multicultural competencies (Corey et al., 2018). The secret ingredients for a success-

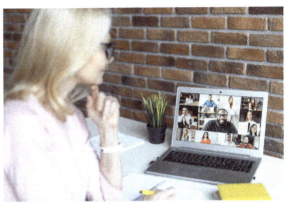

ful virtual group are a solid facilitator and establishing a connection with online group members (Holmes & Kozlowksi, 2015). Group cohesion remains a critical component for all forms of group therapy (Corey et al., 2018; Kozlowski & Holmes, 2017).

Groups have been utilized across health disciplines for decades due to their effectiveness and ability to reach multiple clients simultaneously (Banbury et al., 2018; Corey et al., 2018). More specifically, counseling groups can encompass a wide variety of topics and allow members to learn and grow with one another due to the therapeutic process. Group counseling often falls under one of two general forms: psychoeducational and/or process-oriented groups (Corey et al., 2018). Regardless of form, the counselor must decide whether the group will be open to new participants, closed or semi-closed, allowing new members based on numbers and appropriateness of fit.

As noted with couples and families, logistical issues can be a significant preventative factor in attending face-to-face group counseling sessions (Banbury et al., 2018; Saeed & Pastis, 2018). Online group counseling has been made possible by expanding HIPAA-compliant virtual platforms and increasing user accessibility. Research of online groups denotes positive outcomes and favorable experiences (Banbury et al., 2018; Campbell et al., 2019; Kozlowski & Holmes, 2017). While online protocols for group counseling are still being developed, telemental health for group work is growing and shaping the counseling field's landscape. The next section will provide you with a group case examining various ethical implications addressed in previous sections while accounting for the telehealth format.

Group Case Application: Teenagers' First Session

For this next section, please review these helpful tips to support you in navigating telemental health group work.

- Creating a virtual space that offers each client a sense of safety and validation

  - Relying on security features of the platform (e.g., waiting rooms, camera and chat controls by the facilitator)

- Send materials/worksheets/prompts ahead of time
- Consider sharing screens (for PowerPoint/documents/graphics) to break up monotony
- Consider the developmental and cognitive capabilities of all group members

The eight-member adolescent (ages 14–17) group was established for those experiencing anxiety symptoms related to school experiences. These students did not all attend the same high school but were referred by their school counselors and screened for group fit. The clients were encouraged to uphold each other's confidentiality, as they would hope others would maintain theirs. When the clients logged into the HIPAA-compliant Zoom session, they were greeted in the virtual waiting room with the following prompt to begin the process of supporting a confidential space to share.

Please take a few minutes to consider the importance of confidentiality. Confidentiality refers to maintaining privacy for group members, meaning what is shared in this group remains within this group. As a reminder, your counselor has reviewed with you the only exceptions to confidentiality which involve risk and/or legal reasons.

Consider:
- *How can I feel safe to share with the group?*
- *What promise do I need from fellow group members to openly and honestly participate without feeling judged?*

We look forward to seeing you in a few minutes. Remember to engage with this group with your video, audio and chat features enabled. Thank you!

Per the informed consent the clients signed during the screening/initial paperwork process, no client had access to video, audio, or chat options while in the waiting room.

When everyone was admitted to the main room, after an initial welcome and thanking them for joining, the counselor, Elizabeth, shared that it would take a moment to get to know each other; however, at the beginning of this first session they were going to develop some ground rules for the group to help everyone from the start feel comfortable. She explained confidentiality and limits of confidentiality, emphasized the following to consider for group counseling:

> I, as your counselor, am required to keep what you share here in group, except for some of those exceptions addressed in your informed consent that we just reviewed, confidential. Even though I cannot guarantee that no member will share what happens in group, I ask that you maintain your group members' confidence. It is okay to process and talk about your group experience, but it is asked that each member respect the shares of their fellow group members and maintain their confidence.

The group members then were invited to share verbally or type in the chat the considerations they felt would be helpful to support a therapeutic group. Some of the guidelines included, but were not limited to these:

- Keep all communication public and open in the group (i.e., no private chat options).
- Convey respectful behaviors even when there is disagreement (i.e., no talking over anyone, rolling eyes, scoffing, etc.).
- Arrive on time for sessions (i.e., not allowing access after session start time).
- Keep the camera on during the sessions.
- Inform the group members if need to temporarily step away (chat is acceptable so as not to interrupt if needed).

Once the parameters of the group were devised, Elizabeth ensured all members were in agreement by asking them for either a thumbs up or down on their screen. When the terms were agreed to, the counselor thanked everyone for supporting the creation of a safe space for each member and reminded the clients that if any modifications are desired by a group member, they can bring this to the attention of the group during their sessions.

Group members then revisited the purpose of the group with a brief activity to break the ice. Elizabeth decided to use an interactive activity that allowed each member to be engaged, connect with each other, and share what they hope to gain from this experience. She confirmed that all members of the group had the internet capability to support such an interactive experience, and once received she introduced an icebreaker activity to support the group members to get to know one another and support an interconnected virtual space. In advance, Elizabeth created a digital and interactive Wheel of Names, which included each group member's name. When she clicked the screen, the wheel spun and randomly landed on the name of a group member.

When the group member's name was first chosen, that person was asked to share what they hoped to get from participation in this group. When their name was chosen

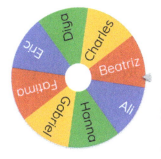

Image 9.5

for the second time, the client was asked to share something they would like the group to know about them. This provided a fun and engaging way for members to get to know one another.

TIME TO BOOKMARK!

Create your own Wheel of Names: https://wheelofnames.com/

During this first session, Diya kept turning off her camera. Elizabeth reminded her of the informed consent and group's emphasized guidelines discussed at the beginning of the session to maintain an active camera through the session. Diya indicated that her parents left her little brother home with her and that he was with her and she did not want to distract anyone. Per the informed consent and the rules of the group, having distractions or others in the room in which confidentiality could be breached was not permitted. Elizabeth asked Diya if there were any other options, and when Diya replied that there was not, Elizabeth gently informed her that she will need to exit the session due to having another family member present that would interfere with confidentiality needs. Diya said she understood, and Elizabeth assured her that she could pick up with the group at the start of their next scheduled session.

Adolescent clients (ages 12–18) are in a major developmental milestone of their life where they seek a sense of belonging through self-exploration by examining personal values, beliefs, and goals (Erikson, 1968). Individuals at this stage of life struggle with understanding who they are and how they fit into society, which may experience an identity crisis (Erikson, 1968). Individuals at this stage struggle with acceptance of others (fidelity) with differing perceptions until some resolution is established with their role confusion. It is not uncommon during this age to experience fears of being judged and disliked. Therefore, providing teenage clients with a safe group space is paramount when establishing a therapeutic space. Not only has unconditional positive regard been researched for improvement of client well-being for people with mood or anxiety disorders (Farber et al., 2018), but Carl Rogers explains the importance of climate setting with the group (Rogers, 1980) and shares how nonjudgmental environments support client change (Rogers, 1951).

Teenagers can be savvy with technology; therefore, the counselor needed to ensure they were utilizing security features to ensure a safe space for each of the clients (e.g., waiting rooms, code words for client verification, disabled private chat features, disabled share for all features, not able to enter the session prior to counselor). As each client was invited to share in establishing ground rules as well as discussing and democratically voting on them, the counselor was highly attentive to inviting each client the opportunity to be heard and to feel validated in their thoughts.

Chapter Summary

Telemental health is increasing in popularity with both providers and clients alike. The consensus for accessibility and effectiveness in outcomes is vastly positive. Synchronous virtual platforms offer a convenient alternative for clients facing logistical barriers and those who may find participating in counseling from home more comfortable. Attending therapy online offers couples, families, and groups the ability to be seen together, even when members are in separate locations.

Technology is not without flaws, but many issues can be mitigated with preparation. Reviewing applicable state laws and licensure board rules regarding telemental health will assist in ensuring appropriate protocols are maintained. Choosing a HIPAA-compliant platform that offers reliability, ease of use and screen-share capability will add to session quality and versatility. Obtaining all necessary client contact information prior to the first session will assist in ensuring client safety. Considerations for confidentiality and tech glitches when utilizing telemental health for couples, families and groups should be considered and discussed with clients during the initial meeting. Having a plan in place for safety and how session interruptions will be handled will help clients to feel more comfortable and maintain session integrity. Reviewing what works well within telemental health sessions and problem-solving troublesome issues also promotes more positive experiences. Lastly, but perhaps most importantly, as with all forms of therapy, counselors should always consider and address self-care needs. There is a lot going on in these sessions; a counselor must ensure they are present in the here and now to support their clients effectively.

REFLECTION ACTIVITY

At this point in the chapter, think back to the exercise offered prior to the case applications. We leave you with the question, how do you do it all? Consider testing yourself and your abilities with being present in the here and now and your ability to be in tune to multiple people at once again. Consider, when out at dinner with your friends or family, taking 5 minutes to inventory as many verbal and nonverbal behaviors of the group as possible. How was it? Are you tired? Consider doing this for a 50-minute session with a couple, family, or group. Anything different you may need to be cognizant of when working in a virtual space?

A counselor's ability to stay present and be mindful of all client verbal and nonverbal interactions throughout the session is important. When working with one client during a session, a counselor can be faced with reservations of the job such as vicarious trauma, compassion fatigue, and burnout. When working with multiple individuals within one session, the energy required of the counselor increases as there are numerous verbal and nonverbal observations a counselor needs to be aware of for all participants. Then add the technological concerns the counselor needs to navigate simultaneously, and you can see how working with multiple clients in a telemental health setting can lead to exhaustion! To ensure a counselor can rejuvenate to continually be an effective helper, it is necessary to check in with themselves concerning the experience and process the impacts. So, let's check in! Think back to your own experiential activity as well as the case applications:

- What did you find most challenging when more than one client/person was present at a time?

  - How could the focus needed during the session impact your ability to be in the here and now?
  - Are any technological preparations needed on your end to support your ability to be present with your clients?
  - Considering the informed consent development, is there any additional research you feel you need to do when conducting telemental health (e.g., state laws, HIPAA compliance)?

- What came most naturally to you for your own practice with friends/family? What do you think will come most natural for you with the client cases shared?
- Did you find it intellectually stimulating to navigate a system and examine client work within their system? Did you find it invigorating to read about clients forming units that were empowering?
- From the cases, what format did you feel like you would be most comfortable with in the role of counselor?
- Did you feel that in any of the cases shared you were losing a sense of control of your counselor role? If so, how do you plan to prepare for this to support maintenance of the role?
- Is there any setting you fear for your future work? If so, how do you plan to prepare for this to ensure you can maintain the role?

References

American Counseling Association. (2014). *ACA code of ethics.* Author.

American Mental Health Counseling Association. (2020). *AMHCA code of ethics.* Author.

Banbury, A., Nancarrow, S., Dart, J., Gray, L., & Parkinson, L. (2018). Telehealth interventions delivering home-based support group videoconferencing: Systematic review. *Journal of Medical Internet Research, 20*(2), e25.

Blumer, M. L. C., Hertlein, K. M., & VandenBosch, M. L. (2015). Towards the development of educational core competencies for couple and family therapy technology practices. *Contemporary Family Therapy, 37*(2), 113–121. https://doi.org/10.1007/s10591-015-9330-1

Campbell, A., Ridout, B., Amon, K., Navarro, P., Collyer, B., & Dalgleish, J. (2019). A customized social network platform (kids helpline circles) for delivering group counseling to young people experiencing family discord that impacts their well-being: Exploratory study. *Journal of Medical Internet Research, 21*(12), e16176. https://doi.org/10.2196/16176

Corey, M. S., Corey, G., & Corey, C. (2018). *Groups: Process and practice* (10th ed.). Cengage.

Duncan, C., Ryan, G., Moller, N. P., & Davies, R. (2020). Who attends couples counseling in the UK and why? *Journal of Sex & Marital Therapy, 46*(2), 177–186. https://doi.org/10.1080/0092623X.2019.1654584

Erikson, E. H. (1968). *Identity: Youth and crisis.* Norton.

Farber, B. A. Suzuki, J. Y., & Lynch, D. A. (2018). Positive regard and psychotherapy outcome: A meta-analytic review. *Psychotherapy, 55*(4), 411–423. https://doi.org/10.1037/pst0000171

Hertlein, K. M., Drude, K. P., Hilty, D. M., & Maheu, M. M. (2021). Toward proficiency in telebehavioral health: Applying interprofessional competencies in couple and family therapy. *Journal of Marital and Family Therapy, 47*(2), 359–374. https://doi.org/10.1111/jmft.12496

Holmes, C. M., & Kozlowski, K. A. (2015). A preliminary comparison of online and face-to-face process groups. *Journal of Technology in Human Services, 33*(3), 241–262. https://doi.org/10.1080/15228835.2015.1038376

Kozlowski, K. A., & Holmes, C. M. (2017). Teaching online group counseling skills in an on-campus group counseling course. *The Journal of Counselor Preparation and Supervision, 9*(1). https://doi.org/10.7729/91.1157

Parnell, K. J., Scheel, M. J., Davis, C. K., & Black, W. W. (2018). An investigation of couples' help-seeking: A multiple case study. *Contemporary Family Therapy, 40*(1), 110–117. https://doi.org/10.1007/s10591-017-9427-9

Rogers, C. (1951). *Client-centered therapy: Its current practice, implications and theory.* Constable.

Rogers, C. R. (1980). *Way of being.* Houghton Mifflin.

Saeed, S. A., & Pastis, I. (2018). Using telehealth to enhance access to evidence-based care. *The Psychiatric Times, 35*(6), 9.

Scott, S. B., Whitton, S. W., & Buzzella, B. A. (2019, May). Providing relationship interventions to same sex couples: Clinical considerations, program adaptations, and continuing education. *Cognitive and Behavioral Practice, 26*(2), 270–284. https://doi.org/10.1016/j.cbpra.2018.03.004

Tuckson, R. V., Edmunds, M., & Hodgkins, M. L. (2017). Telehealth. *The New England Journal of Medicine, 377*(16), 1585–1592. https://doi.org/10.1056/NEJMsr1503323

Whitfield, D. L., Coulter, R. W. S., & Langenderfer-Magruder, L. (2021). Experiences of intimate partner violence among lesbian, gay, bisexual, and transgender college students: The intersection of gender, race, and sexual orientation. *Journal of Interpersonal Violence, 36*(11–12), NP6040-NP6064.

Wrape, E. R., & McGinn, M. M. (2019). Clinical and ethical considerations for delivering couple and family therapy via telehealth. *Journal of Marital and Family Therapy, 45*(2), 296–308.

Credits

IMG 9.1: Copyright © 2013 Depositphotos/smarnad.
IMG 9.2: Copyright © 2015 Depositphotos/fxm73.
IMG 9.3: Copyright © 2016 Depositphotos/monkeybusiness.
IMG 9.4: Copyright © 2021 Depositphotos/VadymPastukh.
IMG 9.5: Generated with https://wheelofnames.com/.

CHAPTER 10

Application of Telemental Health, Part 4
Additional Areas of Specialization

Fredrick Dombrowski

> If human beings are perceived as potentials rather than problems, as possessing strengths instead of weaknesses, as unlimited rather than dull and unresponsive, then they thrive and grow to their capabilities.
>
> *–Barbara Bush*

Learning Objectives

After reading this chapter, you should be able to do the following:

1. Discuss benefits and limitations to using telehealth with examples of specialized populations
2. Identify the unique needs of various specialized populations to consider when providing telehealth
3. Apply evidence-based practices to specialized populations using telehealth
4. Provide resources to assist specialized populations to enhance treatment outcomes

Introduction

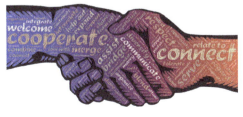

Providing appropriate evidenced-based mental health treatment for various populations requires various skills from the counselor. Converting treatment to

215

telehealth can be extremely difficult for counselors working with specific populations as treatment is not necessarily isolated to working directly with the individual. The use of telehealth for various specific populations requires adjustments to approaches, which may include the family, agencies and community supports close to the individual, connections with medical providers, and engagement with other clinicians. The counselor working with a young adult living with an intellectual disability can feel ill-equipped through the telehealth format. Counselors specializing with those living with chronic pain may be worried as the use of telehealth may promote further isolation. Working with those living with co-occurring substance use and mental health diagnoses can be especially difficult via telehealth as the counselor may be limited to provide a full mental status exam and observed urinalysis to affirm adherence to recovery. Working with marginalized lesbian, gay, bisexual, transgender, questioning, queer, intersex, asexual, and other affectional identities (LGBTQIA+) can be challenging as establishing a clinical rapport may be difficult without the luxury of in person contact.

While this chapter will discuss ways to assist various specialized populations via telehealth, this is somewhat limited as all populations cannot be deeply reviewed. In your coursework and postgraduate continuous education, you will have training that focuses on varied clinical needs across diverse groups. With that stated, to prepare a counselor to work with various populations, all counselors, counselors-in-training, supervisors, directors, and those creating agency policy are encouraged to adopt a mind-set of cultural humility in addition to the expectation of cultural competence. Cultural competence is an ongoing process of education in which counselors learn about the cultures of those they serve to consider ways to enhance treatment outcomes (Ertl et al., 2019). This is a well-meaning attempt to prompt counselors to use culturally appropriate tools for treatment outcomes. Although well meaning, cultural competence is somewhat limited as it is impossible for the counselor to be an expert at every culture. Rather, the counselor is encouraged to adopt a perspective of cultural humility. This concept is a lifelong appreciation of and commitment to learning about other cultures. This mind-set requires the counselor to genuinely appreciate various ways of living that are different from the cultural foundation of the counselor. This requires the counselor to assess their own cultural worldview while working to enhance and advocate for others who have limited access to resources and to promote previously marginalized voices in the discussion of clinical mental health counseling (Hook et al., 2016). The reader is also encouraged to consider the experiences of the populations being discussed.

Telehealth for Specialized Populations

Despite the current trend towards using telehealth, this modality existed during the 20th century as war veterans and those with various medical conditions experienced limitations in personal attendance to appointments (Chen et al., 2021). Traditionally, telehealth was conceptualized for populations living in rural areas who are several hours away from clinics (Chaet et al., 2017). There remained a preference for providing in-person treatment for those living with various diagnoses or circumstances based on type and severity of illness, indicated by level of care, medical concerns, problems within the home, and benefits of engaging in activities away from the home (Hinton et al., 2017). As telehealth has expanded, clinicians have found opportunities to apply treatments via telehealth that were once expected to be in person in a brick-and-mortar setting.

As the ongoing use of telehealth has contributed to the expansion of evidence-based treatments, so too have the populations being served via telehealth expanded. It would seem that providing telehealth to various populations may have limited efficacy based on the unique circumstances of the individual (Singh et al., 2021). However, clinicians from various disciplines have found ways to engage in assessment and treatment of populations who were once not considered appropriate for telehealth services (Jeste et al., 2020). Among these populations are those living with various intellectual disabilities.

Working With Those With Intellectual Disabilities

Clinical treatment of variously abled individuals has been somewhat limited when compared to working with populations who do not have developmental disabilities (Pellegrino & Reed, 2020). Prior to the 1970s, many people who lived with intellectual disabilities resided at state hospitals with limited access to activities and ability for self-determination (Albrecht et al., 2001). The person-centered movement, spearheaded by Carl Rogers, coupled with the closure of expensive state facilities, helped to reintegrate these populations into the community (Carlson, 2010). As a result, many locally based community organizations were created to help those with various abilities live fulfilling lives based on their own goals. Many of these agencies provided case management, connection to vocational and educational programs, assistance to families, opportunities for community engagement, and even instances in which the individual may have weekends or time away from the home to engage in meaningful activities (Albrecht et al., 2001).

The conceptualization of clinical mental health treatment of those with various abilities must be approached via a perspective of equity where the counselor meets the client where they are and on their own terms, and operates within the client's goals and expectations (Jeste et al., 2020). As opposed to viewing the client from a "disability" perspective, the counselor connects with the client from a strengths-based perspective using the client's current skills to help enhance their lives and connect to their goals (Lindgren et al., 2016). When approaching the treatment of individuals with various abilities via telehealth, the counselor may need to have contact with those living with the individual such as parents, family members, or workers at residential facilities (Carlson, 2010). Despite any cognitive differences that the client may experience, the counselor still provides informed consent as well as respects the confidentiality of the individual, even if they have legal guardians to help navigate treatment and life goals (Albrecht et al., 2001). In a telehealth setting, it is recommended that the counselor provide the client and their guardian(s) copies of the informed consent and that the counselor directly reviews this with both the client and the guardian(s). For effective treatment of these populations, it remains essential that the counselor works to empower variously abled clients to make life choices to the best of their abilities (Pellegrino & Reed, 2020).

When engaging in treatment via telehealth, the counselor may engage in evidence-based practices that are appropriate based on the individual's strengths and goals. For clients experiencing emotional dysregulation, who may have instances where they become frustrated with their caretakers, working from a perspective that includes the family or those in direct contact with the client is necessary. As a result, family members are encouraged to attend tele-sessions with the client and counselor. Within these cases, applied behavioral analysis (ABA) is often used to help support the client by enhancing helpful interpersonal skills and supporting family members to create an effective plan to support the client. Within ABA, the family or caretakers work from a behavioral framework in which the client is rewarded for engaging in prosocial behaviors (i.e., behaviors related to goals) while unhelpful actions are potentially ignored in an attempt to extinguish such behaviors (Conners et al., 2019). Via telehealth, the counselor can work with the family to establish consistent schedules and expectations that can make life more manageable and predictable for the client. The counselor can still explore, via telehealth, certain instances that may be triggers for the client and work to identify alternative strategies to respond to these triggers, which may include rewards for prosocial behavior such as favorite foods, fun activities, and so forth. (Lindgren et al., 2016). While these services were traditionally provided in person, ongoing connection with the family via scheduled and adhered counseling sessions and using evidence-based practices can contribute to improved outcomes for those with various abilities (Tomlinson et al., 2018). For every instance in which counselors work with variously abled people, it is also required that the counselor remain in contact with all treatment team members, which may include medical doctors, psychiatrists, skills builders, vocational providers, parental supports, schools, and so on. The counselor should not work in isolation when working with these populations and must consider the family's unique cultural background to enhance family values and provide support for the client (Conners et al., 2019).

Caretakers and family members of those living with various abilities also experience disruptions in various aspects of their lives (Albrecht et al., 2001). The ongoing changes needed to support the individual with various abilities can have an impact on the mental health of caretakers (Hsiao, 2018). Many counselors working with those with various abilities find themselves providing counseling and support to caretakers as they may experience intrapersonal guilt and conflict and even experience instances of microaggression from friends and community (Hannon et al., 2019). During such cases, the counselor may want to spend time specifically with caretakers to allow them to process their experiences of caring for the individual with various abilities. In other instances, the counselor may want to consider linking the caretaker with their own specific mental health treatment to provide full and individual support as needed (Dovgan & Mazurek, 2018). Working with individuals with various abilities requires connections to multiple treatment teams, community supports, and even clinical support to caring family members.

> ### TIME TO BOOKMARK!
>
> National resources for variously abled individuals:
>
> The Arc: Links to services, avenues for advocacy, and opportunities to engage in policy change: https://thearc.org/
>
> Autistic Self-Advocacy Network: Provides an opportunity to connect with providers, engage in online supports, and engage in advocacy: https://autisticadvocacy.org/

Working With Individuals in Chronic Pain

Those living with chronic pain may experience such conditions as a response to a myriad of factors. Chronic pain can be caused by illness, various accidents, on-the-job hazards, responses to assault, and so forth. For those living with chronic pain, all aspects of their lives are impacted (Pohl & Smith, 2012). Individuals living with chronic pain are roughly twice as likely as the general population to complete suicide as they are also more likely to experience mental health symptoms such as depression and anxiety as well as live with co-occurring substance use disorders (Racine, 2018). Many individuals living with chronic pain may experience limited mobility as a result of their pain, and therefore telehealth may seem like a good fit to help these populations become linked with care (Dunham et al., 2021). Considering the potential for suicidality, increased substance use, and co-occurring disorders, counselors using telehealth are recommended to create a crisis plan for all individuals they are working with who live with chronic pain. The crisis plan must include warning signs for major problems, a list of helpful connections (family or friends, if possible), potential activities to help cope, medical and mental health services that are close to the individual, as well as local crisis services available to immediately assist the client (Orhurhu et al., 2020). As many pain symptoms are treated with medications that may have a risk for abuse and even death if overused, the counselor must maintain contact with the client's collateral contacts in the home to obtain feedback regarding the client's use of prescribed substances as well as remain in contact with the pain medication provider to report any potential signs for substance misuse (Doweiko, 2019). Concerns regarding engaging in telehealth may be related to limited observation of potential impairment caused by substances meant to relieve pain. Individuals living with chronic pain or chronic medical issues may have concerns that engaging in the community can cause increased pain (Chaet et al., 2017). In some ways, using telehealth as opposed to in-person services can provide a sense of relief as the individual can remain comfortable within their home. A drawback to using telehealth can be related to the client's own goals if they hope to engage in community activities and to push themselves to be out of the home more. In this case, attending in-person sessions would help the individual to take steps toward their goals.

Those living with chronic pain may experience isolation from others as their physical limitations can have an impact on enjoyment in activities. Despite having love and support from families and caretakers, those living with chronic pain may feel as if their loved ones don't understand their unique experiences (Turk et al., 2016). Within this, there are times when the individual living with chronic pain may feel as if their loved ones don't believe that they are living with chronic pain, and as such interpersonal difficulties will arise, contributing to worsening isolation. As activities are limited and pain endures even during traditionally pleasurable activities, the client experiences a natural loss of interest in activities that used to be fun (Glynn et al., 2021). As pain continues throughout the duration of the day, the client may struggle to sleep due to the pain impacting their ability to relax, or they may revert to sleeping as much as possible to not feel the pain. Depending on the nature of the illness, certain foods may not be an option for the client to eat, and they may experience adjustments in weight. Many of these symptoms can mirror major depressive disorder (American Psychiatric Association [APA], 2013), but co-occurring depression must be considered within the context of the client's ongoing chronic pain.

Various evidenced-based treatments exist for those living with ongoing chronic pain, such as mindfulness-based treatment and cognitive behavioral therapy (CBT; Goodie et al., 2020). These therapies can be adapted for application via telehealth. Using CBT often requires that the client engages in targeted activities in between sessions to help them become aware of their triggers, recognize cognitive distortions, assess how their thoughts impact their feelings, and choose the best behavioral option for a response (Beck, 2011). Targeted activities can be completed via worksheets and tools that can be shared via telehealth. For clients who struggle to use software, which allows screen sharing, the counselor can send CBT worksheets to the client via traditional mail to help them prepare for counseling sessions. Engaging in group counseling for individuals living with chronic pain is also helpful with both in-person and telehealth (Herbert et al., 2017). Group counseling allows the individual living with chronic pain to experience validation and connection with others who may be experiencing similar problems. The group also provides an opportunity for clients to network and review services they feel have worked as well as discuss potential options for additional services that individuals may not know they meet criteria for.

Additional care factors must be considered for those living with chronic pain that may not be represented within other populations. Those living with ongoing chronic pain may have endured injury while on the job, and as such they receive medical care and benefits that are connected to their work. Workers Compensation benefits can be impacted by state laws and expectations. The counselor is recommended to assess if the client's insurance coverage reimburses for telehealth services. Although telehealth services have become more widely used since the COVID-19 pandemic (Orhurhu et al., 2020), there is no guarantee that insurance companies will continue to cover this care. This may require the counselor or the clinic of operation to be aware as to which insurance carriers support telehealth treatment. Additional concerns related to the treatment of individuals living with chronic pain are related to assistive devices that may be used to help mobility or enhance senses. In-person treatment centers often need ramps and access for those with disabilities to easily engage in these services. A benefit of telehealth can be that the client may not need specialized transportation to accommodate assistive devices to then arrive at a facility that has difficult access. Assistive devices for those living with chronic pain can also impact telehealth. For example, a client attending synchronous group counseling may not have full mobility to adjust their camera and microphone, thus leading to their feeling disconnected even in telehealth. Options for adjustment in assistive devices such as headsets and microphones with long cords, easily accessible cameras, and easy-to-use software are recommended, although these are limited to the financial ability of the client (Chaet et al., 2017). This contributes to a greater conundrum in which the client is out of work due to chronic pain but must spend money they don't have in order to enter mental health treatment with an attempt to resume income.

Many cultures within North America value the nature of work and the relationship of work to the meaning and value of the individual (Vlaeyen et al., 2016). The lack of connection to work-related activities will directly challenge how the individual thinks about themselves in relation to their families and society as a whole. With that stated, the potential for increased depression and suicidality exists (Racine, 2018). While counselors are expected to engage in ongoing assessment and safety assurance with their clients, for those with an intent or plan to harm themselves or others, it is recommended that the counselor have updated information and access to local services to better assist the client (Chen et al., 2021). More information on risk assessment is covered in Chapter 5.

Many people living with chronic pain will often receive prescriptions from medical doctors to help manage the pain. A myriad of medications exists, although medications with opiate derivatives are commonly used (Doweiko, 2019). A counselor engaging in telehealth doesn't have direct access to observe and count client medications and must rely on the report of family members in addition to the client's own report regarding adherence to medication as prescribed. The counselor is recommended to remain in contact with relevant others in the client's life (with approved consent by the client) to have an open dialogue regarding medication adherence. There may be potential signs that a client is misusing or overusing prescribed painkillers, which provides an area of clinical concern. For example, clients may run out of medication before the expected due date of a refill. Additionally, those who are prescribed pain medications may be at risk of theft of those medications and may resort to selling such medications to supplement lost income as a result of the injury (Jones et al., 2018). Many states have mandatory tracking systems for opiate prescriptions to assess if a client is engaging in the practice of "doctor shopping." This phrase is used to describe an instance in which an individual may see several doctors who share similar specialties to obtain more medication than would be traditionally prescribed by one provider. This often occurs as the client doesn't inform their practitioner that they have other medical providers and these providers provide similar care for a reported illness (Lowenstein et al., 2020). It is important for the counselor to know their state laws regarding medication prescriptions to enhance reporting between providers. The medication provider can connect with the counselor to assess for the potential of substance misuse and potential substance use disorders, thus connecting the client to the needed level of care based on their symptoms (Pohl & Smith, 2012).

TIME TO BOOKMARK!

National Services for individuals living with chronic pain:

National Pain Advocacy Center: Advocates for those living with chronic pain, provides an index of resources to support those with chronic pain, and engages in advocacy for policy to support those in chronic pain: https://nationalpain.org/

U.S. Pain Foundation: Provides advocacy services and links for clinical services to individuals living with chronic pain and their family members: https://uspainfoundation.org/advocacy/

Working With Individuals in Recovery

Counselors working with individuals in recovery from substances must engage in para-therapeutic activities that may not be directly addressed in some clinical mental health counseling graduate programs. Among these activities include observing patient urinalysis; completing reports to justice agencies, which may cause the client to have legal consequences; and navigating the client's potential ambivalence related to change (Dowekio, 2019). While evidence-based practices such as motivational interviewing (MI) and CBT are often used and encouraged in substance use treatment, many treatment centers are heavily influenced by 12-step programs such as Alcoholics Anonymous (2002), which requires the client to have a sponsor, engage in community-based self-help, and use the *AA Big Book* to reinforce strategies to avoid substance use. The culture of recovery that is engrained through self-help groups has been reinforced for over 85 years. As the 12th and final step of the AA (2002) recovery process requires those in recovery to carry the message of AA to others who are struggling with substance use, many substance use counselors in recovery obtain work as certified substance use counselors (Jones & Branco, 2020). Many counselors in recovery work in clinical settings as they also still attend self-help sessions to help maintain their own recovery. This can be somewhat confusing for traditional clinical counselors as they are advised in the ACA (2014) code of ethics to avoid dual relationships when possible. For counselors who are in recovery from substance use, it is recommended that they prevent dual relationships with their clients even in recovery settings, as this can be detrimental to the treatment of the client, and in some cases can be detrimental to the counselor as well (Doweiko, 2019). When working with individuals in recovery, whether in person or in a telemental health setting, know that there are several options for self-help treatment in addition to AA. Always work with your client and be sensitive to their worldviews and beliefs in order to determine the best self-help and support programs specific to their needs.

While substance use treatment providers work to establish a balance between evidence-based practices and the culture of recovery instilled via self-help, the application of telehealth can serve to complicate treatment. Self-help and traditional substance use counseling have been conducted in person. Switching to online formats in some ways can be limiting to the experience of the substance use counselor who must assess for signs that the client has resumed substance use (Kleykamp et al., 2020). In an individual session in person, a counselor can assess a client based on various aspects. For example, if a client is living with alcohol use disorder, the in-person counselor can potentially smell alcohol coming from the client. If the client uses depressants, the counselor can observe slurred speech, staggering, or disconnection within the session. In telehealth sessions, this may be somewhat difficult to navigate as there can be a myriad of instances contributing to the client being unable to focus, such as caring for children or attempting to care for a household (Lin et al., 2020). To help navigate these concerns, appropriate assessment and linkage with the correct level of care must be made to assist the client.

Conceptualizing substance use from a clinical standpoint requires the counselor to challenge the culturally imposed concepts of "addiction" that exist in popular psychology. As opposed to conceptualizing an individual as an "addict," it is recommended that the counselor conceptualize the client as an individual living with an illness and the severity of the symptoms helps to connect to the appropriate treatment setting (Doweiko, 2019). To help objectively identify symptoms associated with substance use, the DSM-5 (APA, 2013) conceptualizes substance use disorder in the following cluster of symptoms:

- Increased quantity of the substance to obtain initial results (tolerance)
- Symptoms of withdrawal when substances are no longer used (can be potentially fatal depending on the substance)

- Continued use despite the use being hazardous to the overall health of the individual
- Continued use despite social and interpersonal problems
- Instances where the individual has neglected obligations (work, school, relationships, etc.) due to substance use
- The individual uses in larger amounts than initially intended
- The individual continues to use despite attempts to cut down or quit
- The individual spends great amounts of time attempting to obtain or recover from the effects of use
- Continued use despite physical or mental health problems that are exacerbated by the use of the substance

The DSM-5 (2013) further quantifies the severity based on the number of symptoms present. If an individual presents with two or three of these symptoms, they would meet criteria for substance use disorder "mild." If the individual presents with four or five symptoms, they would meet criteria for substance use disorder "moderate." Finally, if an individual presents six or more of these criteria, they would meet criteria for substance use disorder "severe" (APA, 2013). While there are various substances and behaviors that can be formally diagnosed under the category of substance use, these same criteria are used to help identify the diagnosis and consider an appropriate treatment strategy.

VOICES FROM THE FIELD

How have you seen telemental health benefit clients when compared to traditional in-person counseling?

"Clients have been able to access services that [they] otherwise could not due to transportation issues. I have learned that visual assessments can still occur online as they do in the office. It is important to be cognizant of the client's behaviors and observant of changes in expressions and body language. The observation is more natural with in-person sessions. If the client is high risk, I make sure I have a number of a family member that can be easily accessed if the client appears to be triggered. I also have the client sign a telemental health permission form."

—Cheryl Welch, PhD, LPC, RN, Florence, WI

"I am able to reach many more clients who were otherwise limited by transportation or other obligations. Some people who are shy about in-person counseling have opened up more via telemental health."

—Jennifer Meador, MS, LPC, ADC, NCC, CCTP, BC-TMH, Demopolis, AL

Considering the use of telehealth for those in recovery from substances requires the appropriate assessment and identification of the severity of substance use disorder (Wootton et al., 2020). The American Society for Addiction Medicine has identified various levels of care based on the severity of substance use disorder presented by the client. These levels of care are identified, ranging from least intensive to most intensive. It is also important to consider your specific community and the resources available as you navigate options for telehealth versus in-person treatment.

- *Early intervention*—Educational information to those at risk for substance use. Such interventions are often informal and considered for those who are experimenting with substance use.
- *Outpatient services*—Providing individual and group sessions, case management, follow-up with justice-linked agencies, and urinalysis. This level of care can range from those living with substance use disorder mild to severe depending on their drug of choice.
- *Intensive outpatient services*—Usually reserved for those with moderate to severe substance use disorder. The individual may attend 3-hour groups three times per week or 2-hour groups six times per week. The individual will also receive individual counseling. This level of care is often used prior to referring the client to an inpatient treatment program.
- *Residential services*—Usually reserved for those with a history of severe substance use disorder who need to work on improving activities of daily living while strengthening skills related to recovery. The individual will receive residential counseling in addition to outpatient treatment. The individual must adhere to rules of the environment, which may include chores, work, and maintenance of recovery. In such settings, the client may have a roommate and share a communal residence. Some settings can be specified based on client gender and parental status. This is usually reserved for people who are at risk for resuming substance use based on circumstances related to their living environments. This can also be reserved for individuals who have had multiple inpatient and outpatient episodes of care who have resumed use.
- *Inpatient hospitalization*—Often for individuals with severe substance use who use several times per day and who have not been able to obtain sobriety from substances by attending intensive outpatient treatment. Those who are linked with inpatient treatment are often expected to resume aftercare in traditional outpatient settings. If the individual has endured several episodes of inpatient care in which outpatient aftercare was not successful, they may be referred to residential services.
- *Medically monitored inpatient detox services*—Reserved for individuals who would endure severe and potentially life-threatening withdrawal symptoms when stopping substance use. This level of care can range from 1 to 2 weeks. These clinics may provide some case management services in addition to psychiatric

and limited counseling services. Clients attending this type of service would also be expected to engage in substance use treatment groups that operate within the setting when medically cleared to do so. Those who complete this treatment are expected to continue recovery by engaging in aftercare in outpatient treatment, inpatient treatment, or residential treatment (Doweiko, 2019).

Clients may also receive medication assisted treatment (MAT), which often occurs via outpatient treatment. Within this treatment, clients will often receive medication that will prevent the individual from enduring withdrawal symptoms or use medications that may reduce cravings for the use of specific substances. These medications are prescribed by medical doctors and can also be used in justice-linked facilities such as jail or prison (Moore et al., 2019). Many counselors may be trained in traditional "abstinence-based" theories of substance use treatment that advocate for an immediate ending of all substance use on behalf of the client. As a result, MAT and other related treatments such as methadone maintenance may seem counterintuitive. However, these forms of treatment provide an equitable approach to help enhance motivation for sobriety while also helping the individual to navigate various life stressors (Witkiewitz & Tucker, 2020).

Assessing if telehealth is appropriate for those living with substance use disorder can be determined by the severity of diagnosis and the unique needs of the individual (Komaromy et al., 2021). Telehealth may not be an option for an individual who requires detox services as they will need direct medical supervision to be safely removed from their drug of choice (Plescia & Manu, 2018). Additionally, for those who have been unsuccessful with traditional outpatient treatments and who require inpatient or residential services, telehealth may not be an option. Some MAT facilities may choose telehealth options for clients if the individual has been consistent with their attendance and engaging in a recovery plan. However, clients receiving methadone maintenance, especially in early recovery, may still be required to attend in-person sessions as they must obtain their daily methadone dose directly from the provider (Witkiewitz & Tucker, 2020). Telehealth can be adapted appropriately to meet the needs of those requiring early intervention, outpatient treatment, and intensive outpatient treatment (Puspitasari et al., 2021). Within this, counselors will need to convert treatment (individual and group treatment) to the telehealth format. It is recommended that counselors continue to use evidence-based practices during telehealth for both group and individual sessions (Lin et al., 2020).

Navigating potential barriers to substance use via telemental health may require an adjustment to the mental status exam (Busch et al., 2021). Once again, the counselor is limited in assessing the mental status, which could be a sign that the individual has resumed substance use. To assess potential intoxication, a counselor can ask questions to affirm that the individual is oriented to time and place (ask the client to identify what date and time it is while also assessing where the individual is located). Additionally, the counselor can compare the client's presentation via telehealth to other sessions. For example, the counselor can assess for changes in rate of speech, affect, mood, and ability to remain focused on the conversation (Martel et al., 2018). The client can also be asked to engage in urinalysis at various community testing sites or hospitals. Although there is a potential for a client to provide an altered or fake urinalysis, certain tests can be completed to assess if a sample is considered altered, diluted, or fake (Schwartz et al., 2021).

To appropriately conduct clinical counseling via telehealth, the counselor is required to use specific skills that would occur in traditional outpatient treatment. The counselor engages in evidence-based practices while working to help enhance connection to sober supports and links with adjunct services based on the client's unique need (Doweiko, 2009). Adjusting treatment to telehealth may require that the counselor send evidence-based worksheets via traditional mail for use prior to the session. If the client has access to a computer and they have the capacity to download worksheets, these can be used in synchronous software programs that allow the counselor to share their screen and send these worksheets to the client (Kneeland et al., 2021). Recovery is usually a nonlinear process indicating that the client may have some days or times where they may struggle to maintain their sobriety. As such, motivational interviewing can be used to help assist the client with resuming recovery-related activities during instances in which they may resume using substances (Doweiko, 2019). For some individuals, their rural status and vast geographical distance from a medical hospital can prevent the client from obtaining needed medical services during cases of overdose from opiates. As such, many emergency medical providers may use Naloxone as a first response (Rzasa & Galinkin, 2018). The counselor is expected to also research laws and recommendations within their state for the emergency use of Naloxone for family members living with individuals who use opiates.

Appropriately conducting telehealth treatment for those living with substance use disorders requires the counselor to appropriately assess the individual's level of severity based on the DSM-5 symptoms provided (APA, 2013). Based on the duration, severity of illness, and drug of choice, telehealth may not be an appropriate option for all clients. For counselors providing clinical treatment to those in recovery while using telehealth, it is important that the counselor use evidence-based-treatment and link with adjunct services as needed.

TIME TO BOOKMARK!

National services for those in recovery from drugs and or alcohol:

Substance Abuse and Mental Health Services Administration: Provides training and education to providers and clients alike in addition to advocating for policy to support those with co-occurring disorders: https://www.samhsa.gov/

Partnership to End Addiction: Provides information regarding links and referrals for services, opportunities for advocacy to support those living with substance use disorders, and prevention services: https://drugfree.org/advocate-for-change/

Working With LGBTQIA+ Populations

As in traditional treatment settings, working with individuals from LGBTQIA+ communities requires the counselor to have education and training regarding the unique

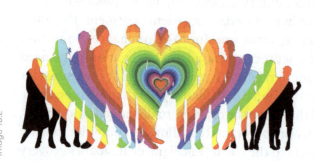

Image 10.2

needs of each community while also using cultural humility to affirm affectional and gender identities (Baams et al., 2015). Working with the LQBTQIA+ communities also requires the counselor to be aware of a lengthy history in which individuals from these groups were not supported and possibly even harmed by clinical and medical treatments (Hughes, 2017). Stigmas and inaccurate assumptions regarding the LGBTQIA+ populations still exist within clinical settings, contributing to increased dropout rates within these populations (Kuper et al., 2014). In the 20th century, homosexuality was a diagnosable illness in the DSM (APA, 1952, 1968). While advancements have been made to enhance treatment for LGBTQIA+ populations toward the end of the 20th century, more work must be done to enhance the counselor's knowledge of these groups. To help enhance your knowledge of these populations, a list of terms is presented below, as quoted from Chandler et al. (2022, pp. 133–134, internal citations omitted):

- **Androgyny:** A person with masculine and feminine physical traits. As the individual presents with these traits, they may not present as distinctly masculine or feminine.
- **Asexual:** An individual who lacks sexual attraction or a desire for partnered sexuality.
- **Bisexual:** An individual who experiences sexual attraction to those of the same and other genders.
- **Cisgender:** An individual whose gender identity is the same as their sex assigned at birth.
- **Gay:** Traditionally used for men, describes those that have a primary sexual attraction to those that share their gender.
- **Gender dysphoria:** DSM 5 diagnosis indicating that an individual has a gender identity not the same as their assigned birth sex. Many of those in this category have experienced limitations in their ability to function effectively as the disconnect between their sense of self and assigned sex causes one or more areas of their life to not reach maximum potential. The diagnosis provides the individual an opportunity to be linked with adjunct services, to assist in gender transition such as hormone replacement therapy, official name and identification changes, and potential surgeries. Having an identity not the same as the sex assigned at

birth is not the focus of this diagnosis. Rather, the dysphoria caused by this is the clinical focus.

- **Gender fluid:** An individual whose gender identity shifts from traits associated with assigned birth sex and traits associated with other genders.
- **Gender nonconforming:** People who do not adhere to societal expectations of gender role and expression.
- **Intersex:** An individual without any medical intervention born with a mix of traditionally male and female anatomy. In some instances, the outer anatomy will not be consistent with the inner anatomy traditionally associated with the individual's interpreted sex. In some cases, the individual may have cells that have XX and other cells have XY chromosomes respectively.
- **Lesbian:** Term used to describe women who show primary sexual attraction to other women.
- **Microaggressions:** Brief and commonplace daily verbal, behavioral, or environmental indignities, whether intentional or unintentional, that communicate hostile, derogatory, or negative slights and insults about one's marginalized identity/identities.
- **Pansexual:** Not limited in sexual choice with regard to biological sex, gender, or gender identity.
- **Queer:** A self-identification indicating that the individual has multiple aspects and identities that are outside the traditional cisgender and heterosexual norms.
- **Questioning:** Exploring one's romantic attractions, gender identity, or gender expression.

Approaching treatment of the LGBTQIA+ populations requires the counselor to reconceptualize the needs of these diverse communities. For example, as an intern, you might have experience working with men who identify as *gay*. However, the needs of this group are not the same needs that are shared by people who identify as *lesbian* or *transgender* (Levounis et al., 2012). While many trainees may enter the field with intents to advocate for these groups, diversity of spiritual practice, political affiliation, cultural connection, and nationalism exist within these populations. Working with LGBTQIA+ populations is not a one-size-fits-all approach but is tailored to the individual's unique needs and goals in the context of their identity, experience, and connection to society as a whole (Baams et al., 2015).

Considerations for potential shared experiences within LGBTQIA+ communities must be addressed when providing good clinical treatment. Individuals within these groups may experience internalized homophobia or internalized transphobia, which may be exacerbated by their experiences and connection to family or society, which may not be affirming of the individual's affectional or gender identity (Swenson et al., 2020). Rates of suicidality among LGBTQIA+ populations are roughly three times that of the national average (Raifman et al., 2020). Additionally, these populations experience increased rates of co-occurring mental health and/or substance use diagnoses than the general population (Goldbach et al., 2019).

It is not uncommon for an individual to attempt to live within a heteronormative capacity, especially if they have concerns of being disconnected from their families, supports, and even work due to whom they love (Levounis et al., 2012). Counselors must work to fully listen to the client and identify how their affectional identity or gender identity may impact the client's relationship with those around them. As is stated within the ACA's (2014) code of ethics, counselors are prohibited from imposing their own values and beliefs onto the clients they work with. In such cases, many counselors may want to empower LGBTQIA+ individuals to live genuinely, being comfortable with who they love and how they identify. While such beliefs may be held very strongly by the counselor, this is based entirely on the counselor's value system and goals; imposing such a desire may negatively impact the client and strain the clinical relationship (Alegria & Ballard-Reish, 2013). Imposing the counselor's own beliefs onto the client can cause a rift in the therapeutic relationship, contributing to increased dropout rates and inaccurate assessment of client goals (Baumann et al., 2020). The counselor must also engage in additional assessment regarding the client's unique cultural and ethnic background to provide culturally competent treatment within the appropriate scope of affirming LGBTQIA+ identities. The client's culture of origin or personal belief system may contribute to worsening experiences of internalized homophobia or transphobia, especially if these issues are traditionally taboo within the client's original culture (Shah, 2020).

Adjusting treatment of LGBTQIA+ individuals to a telehealth modality will require some adjustments from the aspect of the counselor. In most telehealth formats, including synchronous visual interaction, the counselor often has their name displayed for the client to see. It is recommended that the clinician also include their preferred pronouns next to their name. The English language often engages in gendered language. While in many cases the assumptions may be correct, instances in which the assumptions are not correct can be invalidating to the client, exacerbating internalized phobias (Fishman et al., 2019). As the counselor displays their preferred pronouns, this also encourages the client to do so, which allows the counselor to use validating language and speech. The display of preferred pronouns also sets up an environment of support in which the counselor can infer the respect of the gender identity of their client and work to validate their gender identity (Knutson et al., 2019).

Many individuals may engage in telehealth due to the lack of specialty support services within their area. Many clinicians can report their expertise of working with LGBTQIA+ populations. However, they may be limited in their understanding of transgender and intersex needs (Goodrich et al., 2017). Working with individuals who experience gender dysphoria requires the counselor to read the World Professional Association of Transgender Health (WPATH) standards of care (Coleman et al., 2011). This information clearly defines the role of the counselor as well as adjunct services to help the client engage in a transition that is unique to their identity. Some areas may lack clinicians familiar with the treatment of transgender individuals, and therefore they may engage in telehealth to obtain specialized help. With that said, the counselor must still engage in work to find local, regional, national supports, or even online groups (self-help groups, clubhouses, community groups) to help the individual avoid isolation and connect with others. A lack of educated and affirming service providers can be a barrier for LGBTQIA+ populations. Many individuals within the LGBTQIA+ communities have reported their own frustrations with having to educate providers about their unique and specific needs (Levounis et al., 2012). Minimally, clinics and counselors should engage in ongoing continuing education and supervision to assist with meeting the needs of the populations to prevent treatment barriers from arising (Goldbach et al., 2019).

Engaging with other members of the LGBTQIA+ communities can help the individual evaluate their identity and challenge internalized phobias (Bartoş et al., 2014). When a counselor engages in telehealth with individuals from the LGBTQIA+ communities, the counselor must explore resources and supports that are close and accessible to the client. As various states have different laws regarding LGBTQIA+ groups, counselors must research the state of origin for the client to identify relevant laws or regulations that may impact the client. Of course, counselors-in-training will work closely with their clinical supervisors to ensure alignment with ethical and legal expectations.

Counselors engaging in telehealth with the LGBTQIA+ populations are encouraged to use evidence-based practices while also obtaining their own supervision and consultation about the unique aspects of these groups (Craig et al., 2021). For individuals who have experienced a disconnection from their families based on their affectional or gender identity, counselors may engage in family or supportive counseling, if possible, to help repair relationships and allow for improved connection to the patient and their supports. As this may not be an option for all LGBTQIA+ clients, the counselor must also be aware that individuals from these populations may create families or intensely close relationships that are supportive and validating to them. The counselor must approach the client's conceptualization of family from a perspective based on the client's purview and experience.

Evidence-based practices within themselves are an appropriate first start but alone are inadequate with meeting the needs of a diverse group of populations. Counselors working with LBTQIA+ populations must be willing to have respectful and affirming discussions regarding sexual health and intimacy regardless of the counselor's own belief system. Some of these discussions may also require the counselor to engage in additional research regarding medical services and even governmental services for individuals engaging in gender transition as medical treatment and formal identification changes may be necessary. From an agency perspective, it is recommended that agencies have policies that work to affirm and validate individuals from nonbinary and nonheteronormative backgrounds. Ongoing training and supervision regarding the needs of LGBTQIA+ populations will help to translate policy into action by frontline staff. These policies can be respected by and used by all staff regardless of position (Knutson et al., 2019). Additionally, such policies can be enacted both through virtual and in-person environments. When conducting telehealth, it is important for the counselor to have knowledge of local, regional, and national services both online and in person, that support LGBTQIA+ populations as advocacy and ongoing representation is needed. The counselor is expected to engage in their ongoing assessment of their own values while maintaining a perspective of cultural humility when working with LGBTQIA+ populations.

TIME TO BOOKMARK!

National services for LGBTQIA+ populations:

The National LGBTQIA+ Health Education Center: Provides education, resources, and consultation to clinicians and organizations treating LGBTQIA+ populations: https://www.lgbtqiahealtheducation.org/

The Human Rights Campaign: Providing resources (including advocacy, legal, and clinical) to LGBTQIA+ individuals and organizations working with these populations: https://www.hrc.org/

Chapter Summary

While this chapter touched on the needs of specialized populations, once again this is a very limited summary. When considering information about providing treatment to additional populations, the counselor is asked to embody a perspective of cultural humility in which the counselor willingly seeks out such information about those from various backgrounds and living with life circumstances. Several consistent themes are identified within the aforementioned populations. Among these themes is to engage in adjunct services and with families as necessary to support the client. The counselor must work as part of a team and obtain various avenues to support the client. Such support can be completed via phone calls or synchronous computer software that allows individuals to speak with each other. Family and adjunct support can be used to enhance the treatment experience of all populations discussed. Additionally, these populations will benefit from specialized adjunct services (e.g., medical providers). These experts provide unique needed services to each population and engage with the telemental health counselor for continuity of services and comprehensive quality of care. When considering informed consent, counselors must discuss with their potential clients the limitations of telehealth (e.g., crisis, domestic violence, etc.). Counselors work to initially establish a list of services available as close as possible to the client, especially to help navigate a medical, legal, or mental health crisis (Lowenstein et al., 2020). The intake assessment can be adjusted to allow an individual to identify their sex assigned at birth and express their gender identity and sexuality in terms that are comfortable to them (Levounis et al., 2012). In each population previously listed, it is expected that counselors evaluate their own previously held beliefs. Ongoing continuing education, supervision, and consultation are required to assist with ethically serving all populations (ACA, 2014).

PERSONAL REFLECTION ACTIVITY

As each section listed has provided some information regarding national services and supports. You are asked to research supports for various populations within your community. When collecting these supports, try to identify specific medical supports, various treatment programs, community-based supports, and potential processes to link clients to these services. Creating this resource bank will be helpful for you as you work to support individuals within the community. A template is provided for you to work with, adjusting as necessary to meet the needs of your community and populations for which you will serve.

Area of Focus (e.g., Disability, Substance Use, Affectionality/ Sexuality, etc.).	Self-Help Resources (e.g., Websites, Social Media Pages/ Groups, Web-Based Applications, Books, etc.).	Community-Based Resources (e.g., Advocacy Groups and Centers)	Potential Referral Sources (e.g., Medical Providers, In-Person Support Groups, Care Facilities, etc.).

Area of Focus (e.g., Disability, Substance Use, Affectionality/ Sexuality, etc.).	Self-Help Resources (e.g., Websites, Social Media Pages/ Groups, Web-Based Applications, Books, etc.).	Community-Based Resources (e.g., Advocacy Groups and Centers)	Potential Referral Sources (e.g., Medical Providers, In-Person Support Groups, Care Facilities, etc.).

References

Albrecht, G., Seelman, K., & Bury, M. (2001). *Handbook of disability studies.* SAGE.

Alcoholics Anonymous World Services. (2002). *Alcoholics anonymous big book* (4th ed.). Author.

Alegria, C., & Ballard-Reish, D. (2013). Gender expression as a reflection of identity reformation in couple partners following disclosure of male-to-female transsexualism. *International Journal of Transgenderism, 14*(2), 4–65.

American Counseling Association. (2014). *Code of ethics.* Author.

American Psychiatric Association. (1952). *Diagnostic and statistical manual of mental disorders.* Author.

American Psychiatric Association. (1968). *Diagnostic and statistical manual of mental disorders* (2nd ed.). Author.

American Psychiatric Association. (2013). *Diagnostic and statistical manual of mental disorders* (5th ed., text revision). Author.

American Psychiatric Association. (2017). *Mental health disparities: LGBTQ.* file:///C:/Users/fdombrow/AppData/Local/Temp/Mental-Health-Facts-for-LGBTQ.pdf https://www.psychiatry.org/File%20Library/Psychiatrists/Cultural-Competency/Mental-Health-Disparities/Mental-Health-Facts-for-LGBTQ.pdf

Baams, L., Bos, H. M., & Jonas, K. J. (2014). How a romantic relationship can protect same-sex attracted youth and young adults from the impact of expected rejection. *Journal of Adolescence, 37,* 1293–1302.

Baams, L., Grossman, A., & Russell, S. (2015). Minority stress and mechanisms of risk for depression and suicidal ideation among lesbian, gay, and bisexual youth. *Developmental Psychology, 51,* 688–696.

Bartoş, S. E., Berger, I., & Hegarty, P. (2014). Interventions to reduce sexual prejudice: A study-space analysis and meta-analytic review. *Journal of Sex Research*, *51*, 363–382. https://doi.org/10.1080/00224499.2013.871625

Baumann, E. F., Ryu, D., & Harney, P. (2020). Listening to identity: Transference, countertransference, and therapist disclosure in psychotherapy with sexual and gender minority clients. *Practice Innovations*, *5*(3), 246–256. https://doi.org/10.1037/pri0000132

Beck, J. (2011). *Cognitive behavioral therapy: Basics and beyond* (2nd ed.). Guilford Press

Busch, A. B., Sugarman, D. E., Horvitz, L. E., & Greenfield, S. (2021). Telemedicine for treating mental health and substance use disorders: reflections since the pandemic. *Neuropsychopharmacology*, *46*, 1068–1070. https://doi.org/10.1038/s41386-021-00960-4

Carlson, L. (2010). *The faces of intellectual disability*. Indiana University Press.

Chandler, T., Dombrowski, F., Matthews, T. (2022). *Co-occurring mental illness and substance use disorders: Evidence-based integrative treatment and multicultural application*. Routledge.

Conners, B., Johnson, A., Duarte, J., Murriky, R., & Marks, K. (2019). Future directions of training and fieldwork in diversity issues in applied behavior analysis. *Behavior Analysis Practice*, *12*, 767–776. https://doi.org/10.1007/s40617-019-00349-2

Chaet, D., Clearfield, R., Sabin, J. E., Skimming, K., & Council on Ethical and Judicial Affairs American Medical Association. (2017). Ethical practice in telehealth and telemedicine. *Journal of General Internal Medicine*, *32*(10), 1136–1140. https://doi.org/10.1007/s11606-017-4082-2

Chen, J., DeFaccio, R., Gelman, H., Thomas, E., Indresano, J., Dawson, T., Glynn, L., Sandbrink, F., & Zeliadt, S. (2021). Telehealth and rural-urban differences in receipt of pain care in the Veterans Health Administration. *Pain Medicine*, *23*(3), 466–474, https://doi.org/10.1093/pm/pnab194

Coleman, E., Bockting, W., Botzer, M., Cohen-Kettenis, P., DeCuypere, G., Feldman, J., Fraser, L., Green, J., Knudson, G., Meyer, W. J., Monstrey, S., Adler, R. K., Brown, G. R., Devor, A. H., Ehrbar, R., Ettner, R., Eyler, E., Garofalo, R., Karasic, D. H., … & Zucker, K. (2011). Standards of care for the health of transsexual, transgender, and gender-nonconforming people: Version 7. *International Journal of Transgenderism*, *13*, 165–232.

Craig, S. L., Iacono, G., Pascoe, R., & Austin, A (2021). Adapting clinical skills to telehealth: Applications of affirmative cognitive-behavioral therapy with LGBTQ+ youth. *Clinical Social Work Journal*, *49*, 471–483. https://doi.org/10.1007/s10615-021-00796-x

Dovgan, K. N., & Mazurek, M. O. (2018). Differential effects of child difficulties on family burdens across diagnostic groups. *Journal of Child and Family Studies*, *27*, 872–884. https://doi.org/10.1007/s10826-017-0944-9

Doweiko, H. (2019). *Concepts of chemical dependency* (10th ed.). Cengage.

Dunham, M., Bonacaro, A., Schofield, P., Bacon, L., Spyridonis, F., & Mehrpouya, H. (2021). Smartphone applications designed to improve older people's chronic pain management: An integrated systematic review. *Geriatrics*, *6*(2), 40. https://doi.org/10.3390/geriatrics6020040

Ertl, M., Mann-Saumier, M., Martin, R., Graves, D., & Altarriba, J. (2019). The impossibility of client–therapist "match": Implications and future directions for multicultural competency. *Journal of Mental Health Counseling*, *41*(4), 312–326. https://doi.org/10.17744/mehc.41.4.03

Fishman, S. L., Paliou, M., Poretsky, L., & Hembree, W. C. (2019) Endocrine care of transgender adults. In L. Poretsky & W. Hembree (Eds.), *Transgender medicine: Contemporary endocrinology* (pp. 143–163). Humana Press.

Glynn, L. H., Chen, J. A., Dawson, T. C., Gelman, H., & Zeliadt, S. B. (2021). Bringing chronic-pain care to rural veterans: A telehealth pilot program description. *Psychological Services, 18*(3), 310–318. https://doi.org/10.1037/ser0000408

Goldbach, J., Rhoades, H., Green, D., Fulginiti, A., & Marshal, P. (2019). Is there a need for LGBT-specific suicide crisis services? *Suicide, 40*(3), 203–208.

Goodie, J., Kanzler, K., McGeary, C., Blankenship, A., Young-McCaughan, S., Peterson, A., Cobos, B., Dobmeyer, A., Hunter, C., Blue Star, J., Bhagwat, A., & McGeary, D. (2020). Targeting chronic pain in primary care settings by using behavioral health consultants: Methods of a randomized pragmatic trial. *Pain Medicine, 21*(2), S83–S90. https://doi.org/10.1093/pm/pnaa346

Goodrich, K., Farmer, L., Watson, J., Davis, R., Luke, M., Dispenza, F., Akers, W., & Griffith, K. (2017). Standards of care in assessment of lesbian, gay, bisexual, transgender, gender expansive, and queer/questioning (LGBTGEQ+) persons. *Journal of LGBT Issues in Counseling, 4*, 203–211.

Hannon, M. D., Blanchard, R., & Storlie, C. A. (2019) Microaggression experiences of fathers with children with autism spectrum disorder. *The Family Journal, 27*(2), 199–208. https://doi.org/10.1177/1066480719832512

Herbert, M., Afari, N., Liu, L., Heppner, P., Rutledge, T., Williams, K., Eraly, S., VanBuskirk, K., Nguyen, C., Bondi, M., Atkinson, J., Golshan, S., & Wetherell, J. (2017). Telehealth versus in-person acceptance and commitment therapy for chronic pain: Randomized noninferiority trial. *The Journal of Pain, 18*(2), 200–211. https://doi.org/10.1016/j.jpain.2016.10.014

Hinton, S., Sheffield, J., Sanders, M., & Sofronoff, K. (2017). A randomized control trial of telehealth parenting intervention: A mixed disability trial. *Research in Developmental Disabilities, 65*, 74–85. https://doi.org/10.1016/j.ridd.2017.04.005

Hook, J. N., Farrell, J. E., Davis, D. E., DeBlaere, C., Van Tongeren, D. R., & Utsey, S. O. (2016). Cultural humility and racial microaggressions in counseling. *Journal of Counseling Psychology, 63*(3), 269–277. https://doi.org/10.1037/cou0000114

Hsiao, Y. (2018). Parental stress in families with children with disabilities. *Intervention in School and Clinic, 53*(4), 201–205. https://doi.org/10.1177/1053451217712956

Hughes, M. (2017). Loneliness and the health and well-being of LGBT seniors. *Innovation in Aging, 1*, 606–612. https://doi.org/10.1093/geroni/igx004.2122

Jeste, S., Hyde, C., Distefano, C., Halladay, A., Ray, S., Porath, M., Wilson, R. B., & Thurm, A. (2020) Changes in access to educational and healthcare services for individuals with intellectual and developmental disabilities during COVID-19 restrictions. *Journal of Intellectual Disability Research, 64*(11), 825–833. https://doi.org/10.1111/jir.12776

Jones, C. T., & Branco, S. F. (2020), Trauma-informed supervision: Clinical supervision of substance use disorder counselors. *Journal of Addictions & Offender Counseling, 41*, 2–17. https://doi.org/10.1002/jaoc.12072

Jones, M., Viswanath, O., Peck, J., Kaye, A., Gill, J., & Simopoulus, T. (2018). A brief history of the opioid epidemic and strategies for pain medicine. *Pain and Therapy, 7,* 13–21. https://doi.org/10.1007/s40122-018-0097-6

Kleykamp, B. A., Guille, C., Barth, K., & McClure, E. (2020) Substance use disorders and COVID-19: The role of telehealth in treatment and research. *Journal of Social Work Practice in the Addictions, 20*(3), 248–253. https://doi.org/10.1080/1533256X.2020.1793064

Kneeland, E. T., Hilton, B. T., Fitzgerald, H. E., Castro-Ramirez, F., Tester, R. D., Demers, C., & McHugh, R. K. (2021). Providing cognitive behavioral group therapy via videoconferencing: Lessons learned from a rapid scale-up of telehealth services. *Practice Innovations, 6*(4), 221–235. https://doi.org/10.1037/pri0000154

Knutson, D., Koch, J. M., & Goldbach, C. (2019). Recommended terminology, pronouns, and documentation for work with transgender and non-binary populations. *Practice Innovations, 4*(4), 214–224. https://doi.org/10.1037/pri0000098

Komaromy, M., Tomanovich, M., Taylor, J. L., Ruiz-Mercado, G., Kimmel, S. D., Bagley, S. M., Saia, K. M., Costello, E., Park, T. W., LaBelle, C., Weinstein, Z., & Walley, A. Y. (2021). Adaptation of a system of treatment for substance use disorders during the COVID-19 pandemic. *Journal of Addiction Medicine, 15*(6), 448–451. https://doi.org/10.1097/ADM.0000000000000791

Kuper, L. E., Coleman, B. R., & Mustanski, B. S. (2014). Coping with LGBT and racial-ethnic-related stressors: A mixed-methods study of LGBT youth of color. *Journal of Adolescent Research, 24,* 703–719.

Levounis, P., Drescher, J., & Barber, M. (2012). *The LGBT casebook.* American Psychiatric Association.

Lin, L., Fernandez, A. C., & Bonar, E. E. (2020). Telehealth for substance-using populations in the age of coronavirus disease 2019: Recommendations to enhance adoption. *JAMA Psychiatry, 77*(12), 1209–1210. https://doi.org/10.1001/jamapsychiatry.2020.1698

Lindgren, S., Wacker, D., Suess, A., Schieltz, K., Pelzel, K., Kopelman, T., Lee, J., Romani, P., & Waldron, D. (2016). Telehealth and autism: Treating challenging behavior at lower cost. *Pediatrics, 137*(2), S167–S175. https://doi.org/10.1542/peds.2015-2851O

Lowenstein, M., Hossain, E., Yang, W., Grande, D., Perrone, J., Neuman, M., Ashburn, M., & Delgato, M. (2020). Impact of state opioid prescribing limit and electronic medical record alert on opioid prescriptions: A difference-in-differences analysis. *Journal of General Internal Medicine, 35,* 662–671. https://doi.org/10.1007/s11606-019-05302-1

Martel, M., Klein, L., Lichtenheld, A., Kerandi, A., Driver, B., & Cole, J. (2018). Etiologies of altered mental status in patients with presumed ethanol intoxication. *The American Journal of Emergency Medicine, 36*(6), 1057–1059.

Moore, K. E., Oberleitner, L., Smith, K., Maurer, K., & McKee, S. A. (2018). Feasibility and effectiveness of continuing methadone maintenance treatment during incarceration compared with forced withdrawal. *Journal of Addiction Medicine, 12*(2), 156–162. https://doi.org/10.1097/ADM.0000000000000381

Orhurhu, V., Owais, K., Urits, I., Hunter, M., Hasoon, J., & Salisu-Orhurhu, M. (2020). Pain management best practices during the COVID-19 pandemic: The well-being perspectives of chronic pain fellows. *Pain Medicine*, *21*(8), 1733–1735. https://doi.org/10.1093/pm/pnaa195

Pellegrino, A. J., & Reed, F. D. D. (2020). Using telehealth to teach valued skills to adults with intellectual and developmental disabilities. *Journal of Applied Behavior Analysis*, *53*(3), 1276–1289. https://doi.org/10.1002/jaba.734

Plescia, C., & Manu, P. (2018). Hypoglycemia and sudden death during treatment with methadone for opiate detoxification. *American Journal of Therapeutics*, *25*(2), 267–269. https://doi.org/10.1097/MJT.0000000000000692

Pohl, M., & Smith, L. (2012) Chronic pain and addiction: Challenging co-occurring disorders. *Journal of Psychoactive Drugs*, *44*(2), 119–124. https://doi.org/10.1080/02791072.2012.684621

Puspitasari, A., Heredia, D., Gentry, M., Sawchuk, C., Theobald, B., Moore, W., Galardy, C., & Schak, K. (2021). Rapid adoption and implementation of telehealth group psychotherapy during COVID-19: Practical strategies and recommendation. *Cognitive and Behavioral Practice*, *28*(4), 492–506.

Racine, M. (2018). Chronic pain and suicide risk: A comprehensive review. *Progress in Neuro-Psychopharmacology and Biological Psychiatry*, *87*, 269–280. https://doi.org/10.1016/j.pnpbp.2017.08.020

Raifman, J., Charlton, B., Arrington-Sanders, R., Chan, P., Rusley, J., Mayer, K., Stein, M., Austin, S., & McConnell, M. (2020). Sexual orientation and suicide attempt disparities among US adolescents: 2009–2017. *Pediatrics*, *145*(3), e20191658. https://doi.org/10.1542/peds.2019-1658

Rzasa Lynn, R., & Galinkin, J. (2018). Naloxone dosage for opioid reversal: Current evidence and clinical implications. *Therapeutic Advances in Drug Safety*, *9*(1), 63–88. https://doi.org/10.1177/2042098617744161

Schwartz, B., Dezman, Z., Billing, A., Heine, K., Massey, E., Artigiani, E., Motavallie, M., Burche, G., Gandhif, P., & Wish, E. (2022). Emergency department drug surveillance (EDDS) hospital's urinalysis results compared with expanded re-testing by an independent laboratory, a pilot study. *Drug and Alcohol Dependence*, *230*, 109195. https://doi.org/10.1016/j.drugalcdep.2021.109195

Shah, S. (2020). Ethnicity, gender and class in the experiences of gay Muslims. In S. J. Page & A. K. T. Yip (Eds.), *Intersecting religion and sexuality* (Vol. 27, pp. 23–34). Brill. https://doi.org/10.1163/9789004390713_003

Singh, N. N., Lancioni, G. E., Medvedev, O. N., Hwang, Y., & Myers, R. (2021). Real-time telehealth treatment team consultation for self-injury by individuals with autism spectrum disorder. *Advances in Neurodevelopmental Disorders*, *5*, 170–182. https://doi.org/10.1007/s41252-021-00192-z

Swenson, I., Gates, T., Dentato, M., & Kelly, B. (2021) Strengths-based behavioral telehealth with sexual and gender diverse clients at Center on Halsted. *Social Work in Health Care*, *60*(1), 78–92. htttps://doi.org/10.1080/00981389.2021.1885561

Tomlinson S., Gore, N., & McGill, P. (2018). Training individuals to implement applied behavior analytic procedures via telehealth: A systematic review of the literature. *Journal of Behavioral Education*, *27*, 172–222. https://doi.org/10.1007/s10864-018-9292-0

Turk, D., Fillingim, R., Ohrbach, R., & Patel, K. (2016). Assessment of psychosocial and functional impact of chronic pain. *The Journal of Pain*, 17(9), 21–49. https://doi.org/10.1016/j.jpain.2016.02.006

Vlaeyen, J., Morley, S., & Crombes, G. (2016). The experimental analysis of the interruptive, interfering, and identity-distorting effects of chronic pain. *Behavior Research and Therapy*, 86, 23–34. https://doi.org/10.1016/j.brat.2016.08.016

Witkiewitz, K., & Tucker, J. A. (2020). Abstinence not required: Expanding the definition of recovery from alcohol use disorder. *Alcoholism, Clinical and Experimental Research*, 44(1), 36–40. https://doi.org/10.1111/acer.14235

Wootton, A., McCuistian, C., Legnitto, D., Packard, L., Gruber, V., & Saberi, P. (2020). Overcoming technological challenges: Lessons learned from a telehealth counseling study. *Telemedicine and e-Health*, 26(10), 1278–1283.

CHAPTER 11

Counselor Self-Care in Telemental Health Practice

Kelly A. James

> As you grow older, you will discover that you have two hands, one for helping yourself, the other for helping others.
>
> *–Maya Angelou*

Learning Objectives

After reading this chapter, you should be able to do the following:

1. Discuss the importance of self-care practices for telemental health practitioners
2. Explore self-care strategies for telemental health counselors
3. Create and implement a manageable self-care plan

Introduction

As graduate students training to support the wellness of your future clients, you (hopefully) have been introduced to the important topic of self-care. Mental health practitioners have an ethical mandate to maintain self-care to prevent impairment (American Counseling Association [ACA], 2014;

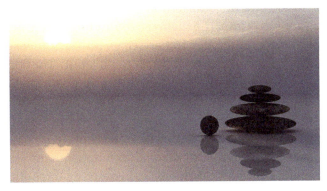

Image 11.1

Scott, 2020). Being a therapist is an incredibly rewarding and fulfilling career, but we cannot ignore the fact that it can also be stressful and carry an emotional toll. For example, common experiences therapists may have during their career include compassion fatigue and burnout. Working in telemental health can add unique challenges such as digital fatigue and isolation. To prevent these negative consequences, it is imperative (and again, ethically required!) to practice proactive self-care strategies. It is also important not to wait until you are working with clients to focus on your self-care. Believe me, I have been there and know firsthand how stressful it is to be a graduate student. Having a solid self-care plan will positively impact your well-being as you continue in rigorous graduate school training and throughout your career. In this chapter, you will explore particular aspects of telemental health practices that contribute to practitioner stress, the importance of self-care, and how to incorporate self-care by creating and implementing your own manageable plan of care while working in a telemental health capacity.

Importance of Self-Care Practices for Therapists

When tackling the importance of self-care for counselors-in-training and practicing clinicians, it is important to recognize that the ACA (2014) code of ethics reinforces the need to guard against impairment that comes from stress and burnout. A primary consideration in reducing stress, managing burnout, and potential impairment is with solid self-care practices. The term *self-care* was coined in the 1950s by the medical community (Houseworth, 2021), with doctors recommending that their patients adopt good health habits such as exercise and diet to take care of themselves. Before the 1970s, these recommendations were usually for aging and mentally ill patients. Then, mental health care professionals started adopting self-care to counter the stress and burnout associated with providing emotional care to clients. Harris (2017) stated, "The belief driving this work was that one cannot adequately take on the problems of others without taking care of oneself ... applied to not just physical welfare but to mental and emotional health" (para. 3).

In 2003, the ACA's Governing Council established a task force to address the increasing awareness of impairment in the counseling field (Lawson & Venart, 2005). The outcome of this effort includes, in part, that clinicians incorporate healthy self-care habits to prevent impairment that leads to burnout. The concept of burnout is not exclusive to the mental health field, as any person in any field has the potential to experience mental, physical, and emotional exhaustion. Warlick et al. (2021) operationalize burnout "as fatigue and exhaustion related to emotionally demanding work experiences. Components of burnout include the experience of emotional exhaustion, depersonalization, and reduced personal accomplishment" (p. 151). The prevalence rates among mental health professionals experiencing burnout are as high as 67% (Morse et al.,

2012, as cited in Warlick et al., 2021) with comparable burnout patterns in counseling graduate students as high as 70% (El-Ghoroury et al., 2012, as cited in Warlick et al., 2021). Have you experienced burnout while in your graduate program? What would you notice about yourself to indicate you were burning out?

Counseling students, counselor educators, and practicing clinicians use the term *self-care* all the time with clients, but do we really know what that means? The World Health Organization (WHO, n.d.) defines self-care as "the ability of individuals, families, and communities to promote health, prevent disease, maintain health, and to cope with illness and disability with or without the support of a healthcare provider" (para 1). In the helping profession, clinicians must take precautions not to neglect their own needs in deference to the needs of their clients. Counselor educators, student interns, and practicing clinicians are responsible for monitoring their own mental health to ensure that clients receive the best therapeutic care. Clinicians providing professional therapeutic services need to be cognizant of their own emotional, physical, and mental conditions and refrain from providing professional services when there has been a decline in any area (ACA, 2014). If a student intern or practicing clinician finds themselves in a state of diminished capacity, seeking consultation from their clinical supervisor(s) as well as their own professional counseling is necessary prior to resuming client engagement. Telemental health professionals may encounter additional stressors that need to be considered in a strategic wellness plan. In the next section of the chapter, we highlight examples of challenges that can impact telemental health counselors in mental, physical, emotional, and social domains.

Implications for Mental and Physical Well-Being

Telemental health practitioners are not immune to the impact of stressors that contribute to higher levels of stress and anxiety. One potential stressor to consider is the impact of technology itself. Technology is an amazing tool that has increased accessibility and flexibility for counselors and clients. While mental health clinicians have benefited from telemental health, there can be added stress when technology does not work smoothly. For example, what happens when in the middle of a telemental health session the internet goes out or there is an unstable connection causing the need to frequently restart the session? This can create additional stress and possibly anxiety when trying to complete a session for a client. Imagine another scenario when you are trying to complete session payments and the system kicks you out, which adds additional time and frustration to the workday. Especially with technology, we cannot predict when things do not go as planned, but we can proactively plan for alternatives when things go awry.

Another potential stressor that impacts physical well-being is digital fatigue. Telemental health practitioners working remotely need a designated workspace that is comfortable and convenient to help minimize the negative effects of digital fatigue. Digital fatigue can be defined as the burnout or tiredness of the overuse of technology as a form of primary communication resulting in both mental and physical exhaustion (Porter, 2022; Tseng et al., 2021). As people in other industries who have worked in front of a computer screen for years can attest, working in front of a digital screen all day can present challenges such as physical strain and eye strain due to the excess of blue light (Porter, 2022). When I started doing only telemental health sessions, at the end of the day my eyes would ache. I wanted to unwind from a full day of hearing client stories by watching a show or reading, but my eyes hurt, and I needed to have some rest time. Eye strain is categorized as computer vision syndrome (CVS) that can affect the body and eyes such as musculoskeletal symptoms that cause neck and shoulder pain; internal ocular symptoms of eye strain and ache; visual symptoms creating double or blurred vision; external ocular symptoms of irritation, dryness, sensitivity to light, or even burning in the eyes (Ferreira, 2021; Watson, 2021) and can even impact the quality of sleep a person gets (Pond, 2022).

The American Academy of Ophthalmology states that the reason for the eye strain is potentially due to the decrease in blinking, with the typical times a person blinks at 15 times a minute. People who are looking at a screen for long periods of time blink half the number of times than typical, creating eye strain. Suggestions to reduce the digital fatigue strain on the eyes has been to take more frequent breaks away from the screen, increase the distance from the screen to 28 inches, and reduce the glare from the computer by wearing blue light glasses, or reducing the brightness of the screen (Porter, 2022). Newer computers have built-in blue light filters, so I purchased a new desktop computer with a larger screen and built-in blue light that eliminated the eye strain and the need for the blue light glasses, thereby removing one of the stressors of being a telemental health practitioner. As graduate students, you have likely spent many hours in front of a computer screen. How have you managed this digital fatigue?

Implications for Emotional and Social Well-Being

As the demand for telemental health has increased in recent years, so has the pressure on counselors to meet the need. The American Psychological Association (APA, 2020) stated that many practitioners indicated that they were seeing more clients and that their caseloads were overloaded, with 30% of those surveyed indicating that they felt they were not able to meet the demand for treatment. Whereas there are clearer boundaries when working in a brick-and-mortar setting, there needs to be an adjustment of boundaries when shifting to telemental health. Personally, I ended up working many more hours a day and week because my desk was always there. I would walk by the desk knowing that I had paperwork to do, so I would sit down to do the work, even on my nontherapy days and on weekends. Additionally, I teach in an online master's degree program that requires my presence in front of my computer for a few hours every day. The outcome of not respecting my own boundaries for my schedule and prioritizing my self-care resulted in the feeling of being very burned out. I decided I had to decrease my client hours and start actively participating in enjoyable activities as a first step to self-care. I created a plan called "Be the Project" that I have since shared with others to support their wellness. You will read more about this self-care strategy later in the chapter.

Isolation is another unintentional consequence that may impact counselors focusing on telemental practice, both personally and professionally. Humans are social beings biologically engineered to be in a relationship (Perry, 2002). Brooks et al. (2020) identified the potential for long-term psychiatric effects of isolation, even if the isolation is less than 10 days. Studies have shown that loneliness has damaging effects on physical and mental health with an identifiable public health issue that creates feelings of shame, unhappiness, and emptiness (Pietrabissa & Simpson, 2020). Abbott (2021) stated that the distress experienced by individuals stems from the social and physical isolation, with younger people being at most risk for mental health concerns and that declining mental health might remain long after the pandemic is no longer prevalent. There are many adverse effects both physically (reduced quality of sleep, lethargy, poor self-care, lower physical activity, poor food quality intake) and emotionally (increased depression, anxiety, elevated stress, and suicidal ideation) caused by social isolation (Leigh-Hunt et al., 2017).

What can you do to make sure that you identify and keep self-care practices *now* as you continue in your program and prepare for working with clients? In the next section of the chapter, we discuss self-care strategies and I walk you through the Be the Project plan I created to support holistic wellness.

VOICES FROM THE FIELD

How has telemental health practice impacted your own self-care and wellness routine?

"Honestly, it has helped a lot. I used to drive, for hours, from one practice location to the next. Oftentimes, sessions began right as rush hour subsided, so much time was spent traveling. Now, I can focus more on client needs, have more time in the morning with my three small kids, and am present to quickly respond to everyone's needs (as there is no need for me to pull over to safely respond to texts or emails). I am more productive and closer to family than ever. At the same time, I am an extravert who is feeling the pain of not physically being around others. That said, I have noticed a rather dull depression since the beginning of the pandemic that has follow[ed] me through to the present. Fortunately, I am working through that while maximizing the additional time. This may include listening to more audiobooks or music (depending on the mood), writing more articles, working out, or just taking a step away to ground myself."

—Matt Glowiak, PhD, LCPC, CAADC, NCC, Bolingbrook, IL

"I found that in the beginning I was not engaging in setting boundaries and taking on too many clients. This was when the pandemic started and so many people were reaching out for help. I felt compelled to help as many as I could not realizing that I was sacrificing my self-care. I have since learned to set very firm boundaries and not take on lots of clients."

—Alice Crawford, LCPC, Carpentersville, IL

"This has been noticeably difficult as it required more effort to maintain a schedule that includes self-care. I use a separate room for an office, which helps to manage boundaries and take breaks as I would while using an office."

—Jeff McCarthy, PhD, LCPC, NCC, Ellsworth, ME

Self-Care Strategies for Telemental Health Counselors

Posluns and Gall (2020), in their literature review on self-care practices for counselors, summarize the importance for clinicians to be aware and realistic about their work, understand the vulnerabilities of the profession, and realize the risk of burnout. Creating balance in all the areas of life is fundamental. Essentially, balance is using a similar amount of time and energy to the different areas of life, being careful to not neglect any area. As mental health professionals our jobs are sedentary. We sit for most of our day, tending to the needs of others, potentially creating negative physical symptoms. Rummell (2015) reported that graduate students reported that they experience more fatigue, irritable bowel symptoms, headaches, and back pain than the nontherapeutic practitioner population. As a result, self-care strategies are imperative for mental health professionals. A self-care strategy that clinicians recommend to clients is a connection to spirituality and mindfulness that help to promote wellness. Christopher and Maris (2010) explained that mindfulness meant, "a type of awareness that entails being fully conscious of present-moment experience and attending to thoughts, emotions, and sensations as they arise without judgment and with equanimity" (p. 115). Probably one of the most important components of a proactive self-care plan is to be flexible with yourself when creating and implementing a plan that works for you. It is also important to identify goals to work toward and keep you on track with your wellness plan.

As referenced in chapter 5, Doran (1981) identified the SMART acronym to write goals and objectives that are specific, measurable, achievable, realistic, and timely. Just as clients benefit from learning this strategy, counselors also benefit by applying this to their self-care goals. The SMART goals explanations and question examples in the chart below support you writing your own self-care plan.

	Smart Goals	Domain Question Examples
Specific	Specifically identify what you want, a strategy for creating this, and the target area of concern or area of improvement; make the goals specific and clear.	What am I trying to do? What areas are working in my life? When will I do what I need to do? Am I happy with how I take care of myself? What areas are not working in my life?

	Smart Goals	Domain Question Examples
Measurable	When goals are measurable you can identify what it is you will see, hear, and feel when you reach the finish line.	What measurement will I use? How many self-care activities do I want to do a week? What is the time limit for doing these activities?
Achievable	Make sure to evaluate your life and have an honest assessment of whether this goal is achievable within a specific time frame or if you are tackling too much.	What do I need to achieve a practice of self-care? Are there obstacles in my way? What are my thoughts about self-care?
Realistic	The goals need to be relevant to your life. When they are relevant, it keeps motivation high and there are better outcomes.	What realistic goals do I need to care for myself? How often can I participate in self-care activities? What kind of activities are good for me?
Timely	Goals should be time sensitive, time based, trackable, and have a deadline to create motivation.	What is the timeframe I want to achieve the goals? How can I keep track of my progress? Do I need different timelines for each goal?

Be the Project

As mentioned earlier, Be the Project is a wellness strategy I began in 2020 when reflecting about how much time and energy was being devoted to one particular area at the expense of neglecting other areas of life. For some, this is work—but for others perhaps it is a hyperfocus on projects, tasks, or a particular activity. The issue is that balance is compromised, which has negative impacts on our well-being. I know I am certainly guilty of the tendency to put work or a project ahead of myself, and I have to intentionally work to avoid letting this tendency get out of hand. Are any of you guilty of putting other things before yourself? Be the Project is a self-care plan to support a balanced approach to well-being, and *you* get to personalize it to best suit yourself! The rest of this section will include self-explanatory practical tools to build your self-care plan. In keeping with the Be the Project self-care priority plan, the areas of focus will be mental health, exercise, nutrition, social, and lifestyle. The worksheets provided in this chapter will support you in the following:

- Identifying challenges and strengths in current self-care plan
- Prioritizing wellness goals
- Completing a flexible plan that targets important components for self-care

Following is a chart to help you get started in discovering what might be preventing you from showing up for yourself in a manner that communicates self-care. These are just sample prompts that can be used at different times throughout your self-care journey. The last column can be used to rate the questions and answers that are most important to you now. This rating scale can help identify what needs to be addressed first, second, and so on in creating a self-care plan. A sample way to use the scale is:

1 = least important to 10 = most important

Let's imagine that you decide the question *What creates dissatisfaction in my life?* rates an 8 for you (pretty high on importance). This rating can help pinpoint the areas in life that can be changed, altered, or eliminated to help create *satisfaction* in your life and in implanting a self-care plan. So, let's get started!

How Am I Showing Up For Myself?

Questions	Answers	Rating of Importance
Reflecting on the last month …		1 = little importance through 10 = most important
What are the signs when I am becoming stressed, burned out, or impaired?		
What do I need to make myself the priority, "the project"?		
What am I communicating to myself when I do not participate in self-care?		
What am I communicating to my family/loved ones when I do not participate in self-care?		
What creates satisfaction in my life?		
What creates dissatisfaction in my life?		

Questions	Answers	Rating of Importance
What are the payoffs of doing things the way I am doing them?		
What is working well for me?		
What is not working well for me?		
What actions am I willing to take to make self-care a priority?		

Creating and Implementing a Self-Care Plan

Now that you have reflected on why a self-care plan is important and what areas you may want to address first, let's look at creating a solid plan. Designing a creative self-care plan can utilize many different forms, such as writing, art, music, movement, and drama (Malchiodi, 2005). A creative self-care plan can foster emotional expression and healing. This practice requires a person to do an honest appraisal of their life, goals, motivations, desires, and problem areas. Making a self-care plan is not about perfection; it is about prioritizing self-compassion by giving yourself grace and allowing for flexibility. This plan is a way to identify areas of life that are not working for you and free the space to add in things that will work for you. Let's get concrete and put everything together to create a self-care plan that can grow and change as you do so that you can create the life you want to live.

Self-Care Foundations

Some basic things that can be done daily and incorporated into the self-care plan include the following:

- Keep hydrated by drinking enough water every day (half your body weight in ounces).
- Get enough rest by creating a sleep hygiene practice that helps you achieve REM sleep.
- Take small brain breaks during the day to just sit quietly and breathe or take a brief walk outside. Smartphones have a "time to breathe" or a "time to stand up" reminder that can be utilized to help get in the habit.
- Connect with your body by doing a brief body scan to identify any areas of tension and stress; you can tighten and release the different muscle groups in the

body and do some full body stretches when getting out of bed in the morning, or any other time when the body feels stiff.

- Incorporate things that cause you to laugh daily by watching funny YouTube videos or a comedy, or do silly dancing in your living room to laugh at yourself.

What other basic self-care practices do you want to include as the foundation for your plan? Take a moment now to reflect on your needs and wants for improving your self-care routine. You can use these questions or use your own questions to create awareness:

What do I want?

What do I need?

Am I satisfied with my life?

What do I want to be different?

What is my vision for each of the Be the Project areas?

BE THE PROJECT SELF-CARE PRIORITY QUESTIONS

For each of the areas, address the following prompts:

	Nutrition	Exercise	Mental Health	Social/ Lifestyle
What do you want this area of your life to look like?				
Is this area something that you want to maintain as is or change?				
How motivated are you to maintain/improve this area?				
Define the action steps you are prepared to take.				
What will keep you motivated?				

I had been working with a client, whom we will refer to with the pseudonym of Mary, on how she can incorporate caring for herself. As she was working from home, she had become lax on caring for herself apart from basic hygiene. Her rationalization was that she would be sitting in front of her computer all day long and no one would see her, so "Why bother?" We had discussed and processed what self-care meant to her, what it would look like in her life, and worked together on exploring the areas in the chart. After a few weeks in counseling, Mary experienced a positive shift and enthusiastically said, "I decided to get up, clean up, dress up, and show up!" As a counselor, it was so rewarding to see that Mary had decided for herself that she mattered first! Each day she reinforced her new mind-set by repeating the mantra *get up, clean up, dress up, and show up!* We continued to map out her self-care plan identifying different areas of priority (self, mental health, nutrition, exercise, and social/lifestyle) for attention. Following is an example of Mary's completed worksheet, followed by a blank version that you can complete for yourself.

EXAMPLE

BE THE PROJECT – SELF-CARE PRIORITY PLAN

<table>
<tr><td rowspan="4" colspan="2">A r e a s o f S t r a t e g i e s</td></tr>
<tr><th>Self</th><th>Mental Health</th><th>Nutrition</th><th>Exercise</th><th>Social/ Lifestyle</th></tr>
<tr><td>**Awareness**</td><td>It is okay for me to care for myself first and gain an understanding of when and why I start to struggle with taking care of myself</td><td>Maintain healthy boundaries and talk with my therapist when needed</td><td>Learn how nutrition helps physical health and incorporate into daily life</td><td>Maintain awareness that excessive time sitting is not helpful to my health</td><td>Notice when I fall into a pattern of becoming reclusive</td></tr>
<tr><td>**Balance**</td><td>Decide to take the 1st hour of the day for myself</td><td>Start a 5-minute meditation practice each day, eventually building to 20 minutes a day</td><td>Learn how to plan healthy meals and nutritious foods that are enjoyable to eat</td><td>Identify ways to balance my work and nonwork life to be able to move my body</td><td>Maintain connections with friends and family by making plans around work and other obligations</td></tr>
<tr><td>**Physical**</td><td>Identify blocks to daily and weekly participate in activities to take care of my physical self</td><td>Process ways to make my physical space more peaceful</td><td>Make good, healthy food at home</td><td>Find three different exercises to rotate to not get bored; start with 3 days a week of exercise</td><td>Enter a 5K race every other month to meet a new group of people and move my body</td></tr>
</table>

		Self	Mental Health	Nutrition	Exercise	Social/ Lifestyle
	Social	Identify activities that I can do away from home that bring me joy	Process with therapist ways to remain emotionally healthy with different groups of people	Plan a healthy meal with a friend twice a month	Join a walking group in town that I can meet with twice a week	Identify enjoyable activities to do once a month with new people to develop social circle
	Flexibility	Recognizing that I tend to be rigid with myself, identify ways to create flexibility into my plan that takes into consideration different challenges that come up and ways to not beat myself up when I am unable to complete the plan for the day. Remember that the most important thing for me each day is to get up, clean up, dress up, and show up!				

Take a moment to check in with yourself and reflect on your own needs as you complete this chart for yourself. Remember, a wellness plan is not about perfection but about creating awareness to support the importance of incorporating self-care into your daily life!

BE THE PROJECT – SELF-CARE PRIORITY PLAN

Areas of Strategies		Self	Mental Health	Nutrition	Exercise	Social/ Lifestyle
	Awareness					
	Balance					
	Physical					
	Social					
	Flexibility					

As graduate students, self-care is a real challenge given the multiple roles and responsibilities that adult learners balance. There are many mixed messages about the demands required for the rigors of an academic program and taking care of oneself by participating in enjoyable activities. It seems the reading and writing assignments never end for students, which leaves less time to participate in self-care activities. Taking a breather or doing something fun can be difficult. With all the responsibilities, self-care is often the first to be let go of in favor of all the other tasks that must be accomplished. This requires a paradigm shift from our need to care for others first to caring for ourselves first. Caring for yourself is not self-centered or selfish; we must care for ourselves to be able to care for others.

- What if we understood self-care as an imperative to being able to work in the mental health field?
- Can any of you relate to being out of balance in any of these areas?
- Do any of you put everyone else's needs above your own?
- Do any of you have small voices saying you are not doing enough, that you do not have time for anything except for your schoolwork, or need to just suck it up and be the super person to get everything completed?

As both a counseling professor and mental health professional, I need to be a good role model to my students and clients. The ACA (2014) code of ethics states that "counselors engage in self-care activities to maintain and promote their own emotional, physical, mental, and spiritual wellbeing to best meet their professional responsibilities" (Section C). If students and professionals are not taking care of themselves, they can cause damage to their clients. Self-care is not selfish; it is not a luxury—it is required to be an effective therapist. Additionally, identifying activities that bring joy into your life, activities that are self-soothing such as a walk or a massage, things that are enjoyable, things that make you feel rested as well as asking yourself these questions to build a plan of self-care: Will self-care make me happier, healthier, more grounded? Will it help me have a positive outlook, help me have better sleep, create a sense of relaxation, or have a sense of accomplishment? Possibly all of these!

VOICES FROM THE FIELD

How do you ensure regular self-care as a busy LPC and doctoral student?

"As a doctoral student and a licensed mental health counselor, self-care and self-compassion are critical for effective, ethical service. I make concrete goals around self-care and share them with my academic advisor and with trusted colleagues who help hold me accountable. I choose self-care activities that are low-barrier and refreshing, but that I will not feel guilty for not completing. Self-compassion is a key element of the process. Scheduling, support, and gentleness with self and others are key elements for balance."

—Marisa Whitsett, MA, LPC-MHSP, NCC, Memphis, TN

Chapter Summary

Mental health practitioners have exhibited the ability to be flexible and creative by transitioning to telemental health service platforms. More than ever, as the professional landscape continues to evolve and telemental health becomes a standard delivery method, professional counselors need to identify strategies for creating and implementing a self-care plan that can be maintained for the duration of life. Telemental health has the potential to impact counselor wellness in areas such as digital fatigue, technology stressors, work–life boundary challenges, and sense of isolation. Areas of consideration for self-care include mental and emotional well-being, exercise, nutrition, social, and lifestyle needs. A self-care plan can start with the individual developing awareness of what is working, what is not working, what needs attention, and what action plan a person is willing to take for positive change.

Addressing self-care goals across different domains in life is instrumental in creating a manageable self-care plan. No matter the benefits, the first step to ultimately making self-care a priority that becomes a habit is to design a personalized and manageable self-care plan. In this chapter, we explored the creation of a personalized self-care plan that included areas of mental and emotional health, nutrition, exercise, social, and lifestyle. Counselors must be able to nurture and care for themselves so that they can be fully present in order to serve others. It is important to craft your self-care plan now as you are engaged in your educational journey to support your success now and in the future!

References

Abbott, A. (2021, February 3). COVID's mental-health toll: How scientists are tracking a surge in depression. *Nature*. https://www.nature.com/articles/d41586-021-00175-z

American Counseling Association. (2014). *Code of ethics*. https://www.counseling.org/resources/aca-code-of-ethics.pdf

American Psychological Association. (2020, June 5). *Psychologists embrace telehealth to prevent the spread of COVID-19*. https://www.apaservices.org/practice/legal/technology/psychologists-embrace-telehealth

Brooks, S. K., Webster, R. K., Smith, L. E., Woodland, L., Wessely, S., & Greenberg, N. (2020). The psychological impact of quarantine and how to reduce it: Rapid review of the evidence. *Lancet, 395*, 912–920.

Christopher, J. C., & Maris, J. A. (2010). Integrating mindfulness as self-care into counseling and psychotherapy training. *Counselling and Psychotherapy Research, 10*(2), 114–125. https://doi.org/10.1080/14733141003750285

Doran, G. T. (1981). There's a S.M.A.R.T. way to write management's goals and objectives. *Management Review, 70*, 35–26.

Ferreira, L. (2021, May 3). *Do blue light glasses work?* VeryWellHeath. https://www.verywellhealth.com/do-blue-light-glasses-work-5092155

Harris, A. (2017, April 5). A history of self-care. *Slate.* http://www.slate.com/articles/arts/culturebox/2017/04/the_history_of_self_care.html

Houseworth, L. E. (2021, January 14). The radical history of self-care. *Teen Vogue.* https://www.teenvogue.com/story/the-radical-history-of-self-care

Lawson, G., & Venart, B. (2005). Preventing counselor impairment: Vulnerability, wellness, and resilience. *VISTAS: Compelling perspectives on counseling, 243–246.*

Leigh-Hunt, N., Bagguley, D., Bash, K., Turner, V., Turnbull, S., Valtorta, N., & Cann, W. (2017). An overview of systematic reviews on the public health consequences of social isolation and loneliness. *Public Health, 152,* 157–171.

Malchiodi, C. (Ed.). (2005). *Expressive therapies.* Guilford Press.

Perry, B. D. (2002). Childhood experience and the expression of genetic potential: What childhood neglect tells us about nature and nurture. *Brain and Mind, 3,* 79–100.

Pietrabissa, G., & Simpson, S. G. (2020, September 9). Psychological consequences of social isolation during COVID-19 outbreak. *Frontiers in Psychology.* https://www.frontiersin.org/articles/10.3389/fpsyg.2020.02201/full

Posluns, K., & Gall, T. L. (2020). Dear mental health practitioners, take care of yourselves: A literature review on self-care. *International Journal for the Advancement of Counseling, 42*(1), 1–20. https://doi.org/10.1007/s10447-019-09382-w

Pond, M. (2022, August 11). *Do blue light glasses work? A science-based analysis.* Axon Optics. https://www.axonoptics.com/do-blue-light-glasses-work-a-science-based-analysis/

Porter, D. (2022, January 19). *Blue light and digital eye strain.* American Academy of Ophthalmology. https://www.aao.org/eye-health/tips-prevention/blue-light-digital-eye-strain

Rummell, C. M. (2015). An exploratory study of psychology graduate student workload, health, and program satisfaction. *Professional Psychology: Research and Practice, 46*(6), 391–399. https://doi.org/10.1037/pro0000056

Scott, E. (2020, November 24). *Why self-care can help you manage stress.* VeryWellMind. https://www.verywellmind.com/importance-of-self-care-for-health-stress-management-3144704

Tseng, V. W. S., Valliappan, N., Ramachandran, V., Choudhury, T., & Navalpakkam, V. (2021). Digital biomarker of mental fatigue. *NPJ: Digital Medicine, 47,* 1–5. https://doi.org/10.1038/s41746-021-00415-6

Warlick, C. A., Van Gorp, A., Farmer, N. M., Patterson, T., & Armstrong, A. (2021). Comparing burnout between graduate-level and professional clinicians. *Training and Education in Professional Psychology, 15*(2), 150–158.

Watson, S. (2021, November 29). *What is computer vision syndrome?* WebMD. https://www.webmd.com/eye-health/computer-vision-syndrome

World Health Organization. (n.d.). *Self-care interventions for health.* https://www.who.int/health-topics/self-care#tab=tab_1

Credit

IMG 11.1: Source: https://pixabay.com/photos/balance-stones-stack-110850/.

Index

About the Editors

Lisa McKenna, PhD, LPC-S, BC-TMH is a professor at Liberty University in the Department of Counselor Education and Family Studies. She is a licensed professional counselor and board-approved clinical supervisor in the state of Texas and is a board-certified telemental health therapist. She is a trained hypnotherapist and has worked as a counselor in community group practices, private practice, and university counseling settings. Dr. McKenna has served the profession in academic leadership roles including department chair, assistant dean, and interim dean, and maintains active membership and service contributions for several professional counseling associations, including ACA, ACES, SACES, ASERVIC, AACC, CSI, and TCA. She has presented and published scholarly works in areas such as identity, developmental psychology, counselor education quality curriculum design and assessment, and telemental health practice. Dr. McKenna is a certified yoga instructor and advocate for a holistic approach to wellness.

Rosanne Nunnery, PhD, LPC-S, NCC, BC-TMH is an associate clinical professor in the Counselor Education department at Mississippi State University. She earned a PhD. in counselor education with an emphasis in community counseling and a minor in educational leadership. She holds a master's degree in community counseling, is a licensed professional counselor and supervisor in Mississippi, a national certified counselor, a board-qualified supervisor in Mississippi, a board-certified telemental health counselor, and a DBT certified treatment team leader. Dr. Nunnery has served as a counselor educator since 2011 and is currently a faculty advisor for the international counseling honor society, Chi Sigma Iota (Mu Sigma Upsilon chapter). She holds active membership in professional counselor associations including ACA, CSI, ASERVIC, and MCA, as well as has contributed to various association committees in leadership roles, such as the ACA ethics committee, the ASERVIC ethics and values committee, and the Mississippi Counseling Association as the ethics chair. Dr. Nunnery has been a counselor and advocate for over 20 years with a variety of clientele and has presented and published scholarly works in areas such as self-efficacy, wellness, evidence-based practice, grief, personality disorders, ethical practice, and telemental health.

About the Contributors

Nicole Arcuri-Sanders, PhD, ACS, LCMHC, LPC, LPCC, BC-TMH, NCC, SAC

Dr. Nicole Arcuri Sanders has participated in research, presentation, publication, and course development for best practices with distance counseling and supervision. Nicole is a board-certified telemental health counselor and previously a distance credentialed counselor. Nicole has been engaged in providing telemental health practices since 2013. Nicole is licensed in numerous states and is an approved clinical supervisor. Currently, she also serves the profession as a counselor educator and supervisor. She has taught online graduate site-based learning courses for 8 years and supervises students conducting distance counseling. Nicole believes in providing her clients, students, and supervisees with evidence-based best practices to support their well-being and their personal experience concerning awareness and growth toward empowerment. Many of her years of experience include working with service members and their families. Additionally, Nicole has worked within schools (primary, secondary, and higher education), home-based settings, in private practice, and within a psychiatric assessment unit. Nicole is a true believer that as the world evolves, clients evolve, and that means counselors need to as well.

Alicia Davis LCMHC, LMHC, QS

Alisha Davis is a licensed counselor in North Carolina and Florida and a qualified supervisor in North Carolina. Prior to her counseling career she was a social science teacher in the secondary setting. She received her master's degree in clinical mental health counseling from Argosy University and is a doctoral candidate at Capella University in the counselor education and supervision program. With over 10 years of experience, Ali has been a passionate advocate for the mental health and wellness of vulnerable populations. She is also a volunteer counselor at The Free Clinics. Ali is an EMDRIA-trained EMDR counselor, providing both in-person and telemental health sessions in private practice.

Fredrick Dombrowski, PhD, LMHC, CASAC, LPC, LADC, NCC, CCMHC, MAC, ACS, BC-TMH, HS-BCP, ICADC, DCMHS

Dr. Fredrick Dombrowski is a department chair with the University of Bridgeport and is the president of the American Mental Health Counselors Association. He has worked as a clinician in the field of co-occurring disorders since 1998. Frederick focuses on the use of CBT, DBT, and motivational interviewing. He specializes in the treatment of transgender populations, personality disorders, and forensic populations, and is an experienced supervisor and director for multiple programs, including inpatient, outpatient, and forensic treatment. As an educator, Frederick is focused on experiential learning through a perspective of cultural humility and an equitable approach to clinical care.

Missy Fauser, EdD, LMHC, ATR

Dr. Missy Fauser is a professor at Capella University's School of Social and Behavioral Sciences. Her educational background includes an EdD in counselor education and supervision, an MA in art therapy, and a BA in art and psychology. She is also a licensed mental health counselor and a registered art therapist. Missy has presented in the United States and internationally on topics related to trauma therapy, art therapy, disaster mental health, and experiential learning. Her professional and research interests include counseling children, adolescents, families, and older adults; mentoring doctoral candidates; trauma therapy; art-based group therapy; and advocating for diverse client populations.

Lisa Giovannelli PhD, LPC (SC), PCC-S (OH), LICDC (OH), ICDAC

Dr. Lisa Giovannelli started practicing as a chemical dependency counselor in 1989, recognizing a distinct need for trauma and family counseling. She went on to obtain a master's degree in community mental health counseling and a doctoral degree in counselor education and supervision with a focus on marriage and family counseling. She has been in private practice since 2017 across multiple states. She primarily serves trauma clients and has specialized experience working with military personnel and their families and first responders. She currently teaches online at Capella University supporting master's and doctoral students in the Clinician Mental Health Counseling and Counselor Education and Supervision programs.

Jennifer Green PhD, APCC #2682, IDS

Dr. Jen Green is an adjunct professor with Palo Alto University (PAU) and Southern New Hampshire University (SNHU). Jen received her PhD in counselor education and supervision from Capella University. She received her first master's degree in special education from Chicago State University and her second master's degree in mental health counseling from Capella University. Jen also holds a degree in elementary education from Trinity Christian College in Palos Heights, Illinois. She maintains a teaching license in Illinois. Jen is an associate professional clinical counselor and an infant developmental specialist in California. She worked in various settings, including private practice, preschools, elementary schools, community mental health centers, and hospice. Jen specializes in working with children from birth to age 10; in pregnancy, prenatal, postpartum, and parenting settings; and with grief, career counseling, life coaching, life transitions, stress, coping skills, gastric bypass support, weight loss, developmental disorders, and divorce recovery. She has a certificate in mindfulness and mindful school curriculum and a certificate of training in trauma-focused cognitive behavioral therapy. Jen has presented at conferences and written book reviews.

Kelly James, PhD, LPC, NCC

Dr. Kelly James is an adjunct professor in the Master of Arts in Counseling Psychology at Yorkville University and an affiliate professor for Italian Institute. Kelly received a doctorate from Regent University, School of Psychology and Counseling, two Master of Arts degrees from Oral Roberts University in Counseling and Marriage and Family Therapy, and a Bachelor of Science in Psychology from the University of Arkansas. She is a licensed professional counselor and supervisor in a full-time private practice, and is a national board-certified counselor, certified clinical trauma professional, child and adolescent trauma professional, certified professional coach, and eye movement desensitization and reprocessing therapist. She specializes in providing counseling to individuals who have experienced trauma. Kelly has previously co-authored and independently published a book focused on trauma.

Amie A. Manis, PhD, LPC, NCC, ACS, BC-TMH

Dr. Amie Manis is a licensed professional counselor and experienced counselor educator and supervisor. Promoting social justice has been central to her early work in human services and nonprofit administration and her innovation in online counselor education. Her research and scholarship reflect her interests in training counselors and counselor educators for culturally alert practice and social justice advocacy, online course design aimed at engaging diverse student populations, and leveraging technology in practice and assessment. Throughout her 30-year career, she has been a leader in meeting the needs of underserved populations in rural and urban settings. She has served on local, state, and national boards, including the American Counseling Association and the Virginia Association for Counselor Education and Supervision. Her most recent appointment was as editor of *The Professional Counselor*. While she has been recognized for excellence in teaching and mentoring, ethics, and leadership, she is most proud of the work being done by her students in their communities and in advancing the professionalization and accessibility of counseling.

Ann Melvin, PhD, CRC, CADC, LCPC

Dr. Ann M. Melvin is core faculty at Capella University in the School of Social and Behavioral Sciences. She received a doctorate and a masters from Southern Illinois University Carbondale in rehabilitation counseling. In her clinical practice, Ann specializes in substance use disorders and co-occurring mental health disorders. She is a certified rehabilitation counselor, licensed clinical professional counselor, and certified alcohol and drug counselor.

Marilyn J. Montgomery, PhD, NCC, BCC

Dr. Marilyn J. Montgomery is a professor of clinical mental health counseling at Bushnell University in Eugene, Oregon, where she teaches and provides clinical supervision. A winner of Capella University's Excellence Award in Scholarship and Research, Marilyn has long been active in scholarly research, publishing more than 50 journal articles and book chapters on topics in counseling and development, is coauthor of *Theories of Counseling and Therapy* (3rd ed, Cognella, 2019) with Jeffrey Kottler, and recently served on the editorial board of *The Professional Counselor* journal as a consulting research editor. She is a past president of the International Society for Research on Identity and is a founder and editorial board member for *Identity: An International Journal of Research and Scholarship.* She is also the founder and director of Wellspring Development, where she provides counseling to children, teens, and adults and values-based consulting to organizations.

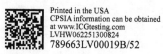
Printed in the USA
CPSIA information can be obtained
at www.ICGtesting.com
LVHW062251300824
789663LV00019B/52